The most com
ask about circumcision.
The answers may surprise—even shock—you!

- Isn't a circumcised penis cleaner?
- I'm told that circumcision can prevent urinary tract infections, HIV infection, and cancer, including cervical cancer in women. Is this true?
- My husband is circumcised. Won't my son want to look like his daddy?
- Will circumcision cause my baby pain?
- My mother told me I should circumcise my baby right after he's born so he won't have to endure the procedure later in life. Does this make sense?
- My pediatrician says my son's foreskin is too long. Is this healthy?
- My son's foreskin is red, inflamed, itching, and uncomfortable—does this mean he will need to be circumcised?
- My ten-year-old is having his tonsils out and the doctor suggested circumcising him as well since he will be under anesthesia. Does this make sense?
- What if an adult still has a non-retractable foreskin?

PROTECT YOUR CHILD'S RIGHT TO AN INTACT BODY. FIND OUT . . .

WHAT YOUR DOCTOR MAY NOT *TELL YOU ABOUT CIRCUMCISION*

WHAT YOUR DOCTOR MAY *NOT* TELL YOU ABOUT CIRCUMCISION

PAUL M. FLEISS, M.D.,
AND
FREDERICK M. HODGES, D.PHIL

WARNER BOOKS

An AOL Time Warner Company

This book is not intended as a substitute for medical advice of physicians. The reader should regularly consult a physician in all matters relating to his or her health, and particularly in respect of any symptoms that may require diagnosis or medical attention.

The title of the series What Your Doctor May *Not* Tell You about . . . and the related trade dress are trademarks owned by Warner Books, Inc. and may not be used without permission.

The authors are very grateful to the publishers and authors of the following works for permission to use and freely adapt articles and essays that have appeared elsewhere:
Paul M. Fleiss. Foreword. In: Billy Ray Boyd. *Circumcision Exposed: Rethinking a Medical and Cultural Tradition.* The Crossing Press, Freedom, California, 1998, pp. 7–9.
Paul M. Fleiss. "Protect Your Uncircumcised Son: Expert Medical Advice for Parents: *Mothering* (November/December 2000): 103, 40–47.
Paul M. Fleiss. "The Case Against Circumcision" *Mothering* (Winter 1997): 85, 36–45.
Paul M. Fleiss and Frederick M. Hodges, Sweet Dreams: A Pediatrician's Secrets for Baby's Good Night's Sleep. McGraw Hill, New York, 2000, pp. 62–66.

Warner Books, Inc., 1271 Avenue of the Americas, New York, NY 10020

Visit our Web site at www.twbookmark.com

 An AOL Time Warner Company

Printed in the United States of America

First Printing: September 2002

10 9 8 7 6 5 4 3 2 1

Library of Congress Cataloging-in-Publication Data
Fleiss, Paul.
    What your doctor may not tell you about circumcision / Paul M. Fleiss and Frederick M. Hodges.
        p. cm.
    Includes index.
    ISBN 0–446–67880–5
        1. Circumcision. 2. Surgery, Unnecessary. 3. Circumcision—Social aspects.
    4. Consumer education. I. Hodges, Frederick Mansfield. II. Title.

RD590 .F54 2002
617.4'63—dc21   2002022653

Book design by Charles S. Sutherland
Cover design by Diane Luger

Acknowledgments

This book has been a labor of love. We are very grateful to all the people who assisted us in its creation.

We are especially grateful to Marilyn Milos, the director of the National Organization of Circumcision Information Resource Centers, for sharing with us the wisdom gained by her years of experience providing parents with accurate information on circumcision. We are also deeply indebted to her for permission to use and adapt several of the professional pamphlets that her organization has produced.

This book has also been enriched by the wisdom of the legendary human rights ethicist John A. Erickson. We would like to express our indebtedness to him for his years of work on behalf of children everywhere.

Special thanks are also due to Billy Ray Boyd for permission to use and adapt some sections of a preface I wrote for his excellent book, *Circumcision Exposed: Rethinking a Medical and Cultural Tradition.* With equal gratitude, we would like to thank Dr. Mark David Reiss for permission to reproduce examples of his beautiful writings.

Special thanks are also due to our editor at Warner Books, John Aherne, as well as to his editorial staff for all their hard work and for their expert advice and judicious assistance.

Contents

Introduction

Babies are a miracle. They arrive into the world complete and perfect with all their functional parts. It is our job as parents, teachers, and concerned human beings to guide them in their growth and development so that they can become intelligent, compassionate, responsible, and healthy individuals in mind, body, and spirit.

A baby is born into an imperfect world, yet he or she is pure and full of trust. A baby's wants and needs are simple. A baby needs nourishment—not only physical, but emotional nourishment. A baby wants to be held and hugged and loved and kissed and touched, to hear music—soothing and gentle sounds—like those produced by a loving human voice.

As a young medical student in the 1960s, I was excited about entering a profession that would enable me to help, comfort, and protect babies. And yet, ironically, one of the things I was required to learn as a medical student was the technique of performing the surgical procedure of male circumcision. It was not difficult to learn how to do this procedure, and I rapidly became expert at removing the foreskin from a newborn. I was able to do circumcisions in a very short amount of time—four or five minutes. I did this at the parents' request, and yet I was oblivious to the infant's cry. I had been taught that circumcision was just a routine procedure—something that was just *done* to little boys when they were born. I naturally assumed that there were sound medical reasons for the surgery. I was an expert at cutting off the foreskin, but I knew nothing about the foreskin.

I had little understanding about what its functions were. I was ignorant of how this surgery would affect a male for the rest of his life.

After several years into my pediatrics career, and after having performed perhaps a hundred circumcisions, a strange thing happened to me: I became aware of the suffering, pain, and trauma that a baby experiences when he is circumcised. Somehow, I had previously managed to put the baby's trauma out of my consciousness. I now realized that every baby I circumcised cried in terror and pain, and that I had failed to respond to their pain. I also realized that I was harming rather than helping babies. I then decided that I would henceforth be on their side; as a doctor, my job was to protect babies, not harm them. After all, I had taken an oath to "first do no harm."

That was when I began to study the foreskin and how nature intended the intact penis to look and function. Through diligent research, I learned how the foreskin is unlike any other part of the human body. I learned that the foreskin has a great number of special and important functions. I learned that the foreskin provides its owner with a lifetime of benefits and advantages.

Another thing that I quickly learned was that circumcision is an emotionally charged subject that most people—and this includes doctors—are reluctant to discuss openly, let alone objectively. I should know: As a pediatrician, I have been on the front line of the circumcision debate for more than thirty years.

Although I have provided information on circumcision for expectant couples for years, it long ago became clear to me that the decision about whether or not to circumcise a boy is seldom made on the basis of medical facts. Even when parents think that they know the medical facts about circumcision, I find that most of what they believe is incorrect. Most of this incorrect information comes from friends, relatives, newspaper headlines, magazines, and talk radio. In other words, it comes from non-professionals and journalists rather than from informed and objective doctors.

The sad truth is that doctors can be poor sources of information as well! Most doctors today know very little about circumcision. They know even less about the anatomy and functions of the foreskin. How can doctors give parents accurate advice on circumcision if they are ignorant of the facts about the body part that is being cut off? Thankfully, there is a large body of medical literature that does provide all the facts you will ever need to help you make the right decision for your son.

In the United States at present, more than two million baby boys are born each year. The parents of nearly every one of these newborns will be faced with what is probably the most unnecessarily distressing decision they will ever make: whether or not to circumcise their newborn baby. In an ideal world, parents would simply enjoy the arrival of a new child without such worries, but because they are forced to make this traumatic decision, the birth of a baby boy can be fraught with anxiety, self-doubt, and confusion. Accurate, up-to-date, and thorough information about circumcision would help ease the tension, but where can parents get this help? Where can parents get the answers they deserve?

Astonishingly, doctors give parents almost *no* accurate or useful information on the subject! In one recent study,[1] almost 40 percent of American parents of newborn boys believed that doctors had failed to provide them with *enough* information about circumcision. Even more worrying, 46 percent of the parents reported that doctors failed to give them *any* medical information about circumcision. Not surprisingly, this survey documented the fact that 82.8 percent of parents in the first six months of their baby boy's life regretted the decision they made about circumcision. That is an alarming statistic.

Why do doctors routinely fail to provide adequate and unbiased information about circumcision to the parents who need it most? You will be astonished to learn that there are a variety of complex reasons for this failure. You see, even though doctors who advise parents about circumcision are *required* to be experts on the subject and are supposed to keep up with the latest research, most of these doctors are dangerously ignorant.

Most doctors who discuss circumcision with parents rely on outdated, incomplete, or disproved material. The sad thing is that most doctors form their opinions about circumcision from uninformed and misguided medical school professors as well as from the same source as most parents: from newspaper headlines, magazine articles, and radio talk show hosts of questionable reliability and dubious credentials. The opinions about circumcision that doctors and other health care writers have may also be strongly influenced by more insidious forces, such as personal bias, misdirected religious zealotry, prejudice, identity anxieties, sexual insecurities, male rivalry, and fear.

There does exist a very large body of excellent scientific literature on circumcision, but the unpleasant truth is that most doctors are simply unable to find the time to read it for themselves. Even more worrying: Accurate information about the foreskin itself is almost always missing from discussions about circumcision. How can parents make a rational decision about circumcision when they are told nothing about the part that will be cut off?

The mass circumcision campaigns of the past few decades have resulted in pandemic ignorance about the remarkable structure called the foreskin and its versatile role in human health and sexuality. Ignorance and false information about the foreskin and about the genuine indications for circumcision are rampant in American medical education and practice. It is embarrassing to report that most American medical textbooks depict the human penis, without explanation, as circumcised—as if it were so by nature. This is as scientifically unacceptable and as misleading as it would be to have a textbook illustration of a human hand that omitted the index finger. It is little wonder that the majority of doctors give parents false information or even no information at all.

Even so, circumcision is probably the most controversial subject in American medicine today. It seems as though almost everyone has strong opinions on the subject. The fact that you are reading this book indicates that you are strongly motivated to move beyond *opinions* and are determined to look for competent guidance and trustworthy answers. Chances are that you take your own health, and that of your loved ones, very much to heart. If you're looking for the best medical evidence that will guide you to take the most ethical, responsible, rational, and *scientific* course of action, we invite you to weigh the facts and see how circumcision would effect the lifelong health and well-being of your child. If, on the other hand, you protected your baby boy from circumcision when he was born, we invite you to educate yourself so that you can continue to protect your son from ignorant or misguided medical personnel who mistakenly think that there is something wrong with his penis and that it needs to be circumcised.

If you're like me, you would rather avoid reading a lot of opinions by doctors who have already made up their minds. You want hard facts. The hard facts, in the case of circumcision, are available and plentiful. The facts about the proper care of the intact penis are also available and widely practiced by civilized nations all over the world. You will also find, as I have, that this is high-level science. There are more than enough medical facts to give you a range of strategies to protect your son from unnecessary surgery. After all, even if your mind is already made up one way or the other, you will have to admit that it is always more reasonable to avoid unnecessary surgery.

One area where people have a lot of misperceptions is the *rate* of circumcision. What percentage of males are circumcised today? We are not a society of nudists, so most doctors and parents have no real idea what the frequency of circumcision is in our country. Most adult American males base their assumptions about the frequency of circumcision on their recollections of what they observed in the locker room back in high school. Medical practice has changed a lot since those days, but most men are simply unaware of this. Accurate, up-to-date information is important because, for better or for worse, most middle-class Americans want to conform to what everyone else is doing. Most doctors who recommend circumcision and most parents whose sons are subjected to circumcision assume that *all* males in America are circumcised. Some parents even believe that circumcision is required by law.[2] Furthermore, many Americans assume that all males throughout the world are circumcised. Many naturally believe that circumcision has always been practiced in the United States. As it happens, all of these beliefs are false.

The fact is that in 1998 (the latest year for which we have statistics), 1.1 million healthy newborn American baby boys were systematically subjected to circumcision.[3] This may seem like an awful lot—and it is!—but this represents a remarkable fall in the rate of circumcision since large-scale routine neonatal circumcision began in the 1950s. In fact, the rate continues to drop dramatically. The average rate was close to 90 percent during the 1970s, but today it is just about 50 percent nationally. In the western quarter of the United States, the rate is less than 30 percent and falling. Rather than all or even most baby boys being circumcised today, very few, in fact, are being circumcised.

Many Americans are surprised to learn that male circumcision is extremely rare outside the United States. It is found primarily in Third World Muslim countries—such as Iran, Saudi Arabia, and Somalia—in Israel among Jews, in some primitive African tribes, and among some Australian and New Guinea aborigines. These peoples circumcise males for supposed religious reasons or as a painful rite of passage. Some of them also circumcise females or perform other blood rituals such as knocking out teeth, ritual scarification, lip distension, and other bodily mutilations.

Routine circumcision is unheard of among the civilizations of continental Europe, Great Britain, South America, and non-Muslim Asia. Most Europeans—including European doctors—are shocked to learn that routine circumcision goes on in the United States. Most refuse to believe that such a thing is possible in a civilized, Western country.

Another fact that you should know is that routine circumcision has not always been practiced in the United States. It was only after World War II that most American hospitals instituted neonatal circumcision as a routine procedure. Prior to that, the vast majority of American boys were just like European boys in this respect.

When American parents learn these facts, they have even more questions. Nearly every day, parents come into my office, or call me on the telephone, asking very intelligent questions about circumcision. The most common are:

- How is it possible for American doctors to have such a radically different perspective on circumcision from European doctors?
- Are European males more healthy or less healthy than American males because of this difference?

- If circumcision is nonexistent in Europe, how and why did circumcision begin in the United States?
- Is circumcision really medically necessary?
- Does circumcision have any benefits or drawbacks?
- What surgical risks does the operation pose to my baby?
- What actually happens to the penis and to the baby during a circumcision?
- Will circumcision cause my baby pain and discomfort?
- Does my baby's penis need to match his father's penis?
- What is the foreskin?
- What are the real medical facts about circumcision?
- If I protect my son from circumcision, how should I take care of his penis?

These are among the many questions that concerned parents ask. We will be answering these and many other questions in the following chapters. My coauthor and I are proud to say that we have thoroughly examined *all* the scientific literature on circumcision. This book is the culmination of nearly four decades of research. In my years as a pediatrician, I have devoted much of my career to providing expectant parents with accurate, up-to-date information on circumcision, which my staff and I strongly believe that parents deserve. I have always found that parents are very eager to learn more. After all, circumcision is a very difficult issue. Getting the answers that parents need always results in greater confidence and in happier outcomes for babies.

Whether you already have a son, are expecting a son, or just want more information, we invite you to read on and learn all the medical facts about circumcision and the care of the intact penis. Notice that I write "intact" instead of "uncircumcised." We would never call normal women "unmastectomized" or "unclitoridectomized." We call them "intact" because that is what they are. Therefore, we should call men who possess a complete penis what they are: "intact." "Uncircumcised" is an unscientific, unhelpful, useless, and confusing term because it uses terminology normally reserved for abnormality to name a normal body part. Let us avoid confusion and stick to science.

I congratulate you for reading this book. This means that you are motivated to find objective and scientific answers to one of the hardest questions that faces American parents today. I invite all parents to embark upon a journey of discovery, knowledge, and improved health for their sons. I am proud to provide you with the information that you need to be the very best parent you can be. You deserve this respect, and so do your sons.

In the spirit of science and compassion, I urge you to read this book with an open mind. It may well change the entire way you view circumcision. If you have already made up your mind about circumcision, that is fine. You are entitled to your opinion. I will not try to change your mind. I would, however, like to ask you the following question: If there were a piece of information about circumcision that would make you change your mind, would you want to be aware of it? If not, why not?

You have nothing to lose by learning as much about circumcision as you can. Whatever your feelings about circumcision, you deserve to know exactly what is being cut off, the biological functions of the foreskin, how the circumcision surgery is actually carried out, and what risks and disadvantages it holds. Of equal importance, you deserve an honest and objective scientific appraisal of the medical literature about circumcision. Finally, all parents confronted with the problem of circumcision need to know what alternatives there are. These are the basic principles of informed consent. In the following chapters, I will provide you with all the known facts about circumcision. Knowledge is power, and this power will help you become a more informed and therefore a *better* parent.

WHAT YOUR DOCTOR MAY
NOT TELL YOU ABOUT
CIRCUMCISION

Chapter One

• • •

What Is the Foreskin?
Anatomical and Physiological Facts That Your Doctor May Not Know

The prepuce is a common anatomical structure of the male and female external genitalia of all human and non-human primates; it has been present in primates for at least 65 million years, and is likely to be over 100 million years old, based on its commonality as an anatomical feature in mammals.[1]

Christopher J. Cold, M.D., and John R. Taylor, M.D.

WHAT IS THE FORESKIN?

The foreskin—also known as the *prepuce*—is the flexible, double-layered sheath of specialized skin that covers and protects the *glans* (or head) of the normal penis. The foreskin is a uniquely specialized, sensitive, and functional organ of touch. No other part of the body serves the same purpose.

The foreskin is an integral and important part of the skin system of the penis. It is a complex and sophisticated structure

1

with many interesting and unique properties. No other part of the body's skin covering duplicates the amazing design and functional possibilities of the foreskin. Among the many interesting features of the foreskin is the fact that it is highly elastic, entirely devoid of any subcutaneous fat, and lined with a sheet of smooth muscle.

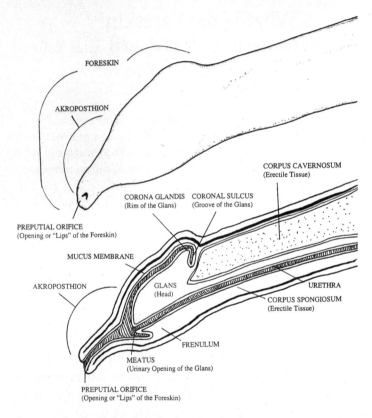

The foreskin is more than just skin; it is a complex, highly mobile, and beautifully engineered organ composed of an intricate web of blood vessels, muscle, and nerves. In fact, the foreskin contains about 240 feet of nerve fibers and tens of thousands of specialized erotogenic nerve endings of various types, which can feel the slightest pressure, the lightest touch, the smallest motion, the subtlest changes in temperature, and the finest gradations in texture.

Nature has designed the delicate glans (commonly called the head of the penis) to be an *internal* organ. In the normal, intact penis, the glans is a glistening, rich red or purple color. The foreskin protects the glans and keeps it in excellent condition.

In many ways, the foreskin is just like the eyelid. It covers, cleans, and protects the glans just as the eyelid covers, cleans, and protects the eye. Also, just as the eyelid can open and close to uncover the eye, so the foreskin can open to reveal the delicate glans. The foreskin's inside fold is lined with a smooth red tissue called *mucous membrane.* This type of tissue is also found lining the lips, the inside of the mouth, and the inner fold of the eyelid. The foreskin's soothing inner fold gently keeps the surface of the glans healthy, clean, shiny, warm, soft, moist, and sensitive.

WHAT IS THE TUBULAR TIP OF THE FORESKIN CALLED?

The *akroposthion* is the useful name that the ancient Greeks gave to the tubular, tapered "neck" of the foreskin that extends beyond the glans (head).[2] The akroposthion smoothly extends beyond the glans, forming a soft, tapered, tubular sheath.

This akroposthion of the foreskin functions as an extension of the urethra and conveys urine from the *meatus* (the urinary opening in the glans) to the outside world. The akroposthion varies in length between individuals. In childhood, it can represent at least half the length of the penis. Some boys have a foreskin that extends an inch or more beyond the glans. In other males, the akroposthion can be almost nonexistent, in which case the meatus and the surrounding portion of the glans may be exposed. Whatever the case, all lengths are normal.

HOW BIG IS THE FORESKIN?

The foreskin is the largest part of the skin system of the penis. It covers and usually extends far beyond the glans before folding under itself to its circumferential point of attachment just behind the *corona* (the rim of the glans). The foreskin is, therefore, a double-layered organ. Its true length is twice the length of its external fold and comprises as much as 80 percent or more of the penile skin covering.[3] In children, the foreskin often runs to impressive lengths, frequently representing over three quarters of the length of the penis.

If the average adult foreskin were unfolded and laid flat and unstretched, it would be approximately the size of a 3 x 5 index card. Moderately stretched, it would entirely cover a man's forehead or the back of his hand and fingers. That's a lot of skin!

DOES THE FORESKIN HAVE MUSCLES?

Yes. The foreskin, like the rest of the penile skin system and scrotum, is lined with the *dartos muscle sheet.* It is also called the *peripenic muscle* because it wraps around (*peri*) the penis (*-penic*). This remarkably powerful muscle is composed of smooth muscle fibers that run parallel to the shaft of the penis.[4] The dartos muscle is involuntary and highly responsive. It contracts and relaxes in response to touch, temperature, and sexual excitement.

The dartos muscle is always in a state of *tonus,* or partial contraction—a condition of tension or readiness to contract or relax. The contractions of the dartos muscle are slow, sustained, and may produce great force, such as in cold temperatures.

WHAT ARE EVERSION AND REVERSION?

Eversion is the natural mechanical process by which the lips of the foreskin open and allow the foreskin to unroll and slide down the shaft of the penis to reveal the glans. When fully everted, the inner fold of the foreskin that embraces the glans is turned inside-out and moves along the shaft of the penis.

Reversion is the reverse process that rolls the foreskin back up the shaft of the penis to cover the glans. Following eversion, the elastic skin system of the penis will usually have a tendency to return to its normal position, re-covering the glans and pursing the lips of the foreskin. Reversion is accomplished through the springlike action of the *frenulum.*

WHAT IS UNIQUE ABOUT THE PREPUTIAL ORIFICE?

At the very end of the foreskin lies the rose-colored *preputial orifice,* also known as the lips of the foreskin. Here, the muscle fibers form a kind of sphincter that ensures optimum protection of the urinary tract from contaminants of all kinds.[5] This functions similarly to the sphincter that closes and purses the lips of your mouth.

In terms of sensitivity, the lips of the foreskin are probably even more sensitive than the lips of the mouth in their ability to detect subtle differences in temperature, pressure, motion, and touch. The orifice remains closed most of the time, but can open up to allow the passage of urine. Thanks to its highly elas-

tic nature, the preputial sphincter can easily and comfortably dilate over ten times its normal diameter to allow the glans to protrude.

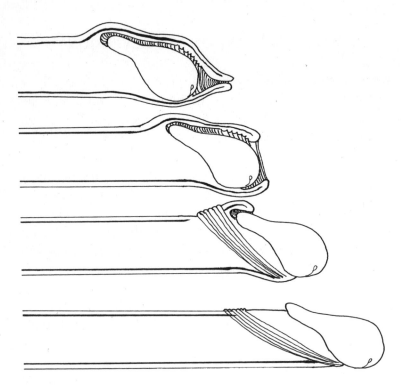

Eversion of the Foreskin

WHAT IS SPECIAL ABOUT THE
INNER SURFACE OF THE FORESKIN?

Like the undersurface of the eyelids or the inside of the cheek,
the undersurface of the foreskin is lined with a rich red-colored
mucous membrane. It is divided into two distinct zones: the

smooth mucosa and the *ridged mucosa*. The smooth mucosa lies against the glans penis. Here, researchers have discovered apocrine and ectopic sebaceous glands that secrete emollients, lubricants, and protective antibodies.[6] Similar glands are found in the eyelids and mouth.

WHAT DOES THE RIDGED MUCOSA DO?

Adjacent to the smooth mucosa and just behind the lips of the foreskin is the ridged mucosa. This exquisitely sensitive structure consists of tightly pleated concentric bands, like the elastic bands at the top of a sock. These expandable pleats arise from the frenulum and encircle the inner lining of the foreskin. They allow the lips of the foreskin to open and roll back, exposing the glans. The ridged mucosa also gives the foreskin its characteristic taper.

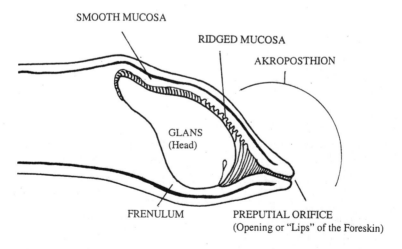

Cross-section of the Penis

The ridged mucosa is a highly vascular zone of specialized sensory tissue containing a dense concentration of specialized erotogenic nerve receptors.[7] Eversion and reversion of the foreskin during erection and sexual play cause the pleats of the ridged mucosa to expand and contract like the bellows of an accordion. This movement allows every surface of the pleats to come in contact with the rim of the glans. The unfolding and refolding of the ridged mucosa over the glans allows all the erotogenic nerve endings to be stimulated, increasing sexual pleasure. If the foreskin is fully everted, the ridged mucosa will be repositioned around the shaft of the penis.

WHAT IS THE SMOOTH MUCOSA?

The last segment of the internal foreskin is the smooth mucosa, which extends from the last ridge of the ridged mucosa to the point of attachment at the coronal sulcus. The surface of this segment is composed of stratified squamous epithelial mucous membrane.

WHAT IS THE FRENULUM?

On the underside of the glans, the foreskin's point of attachment to the body of the penis is the muscular, bandlike ligament called the frenulum. If you turn your lower lip down, or your upper lip up, you will see a similar ligament that serves a very similar function in holding the lips in place. The tongue also has a frenulum that holds it in place. The frenulum functions as a spring, holding the foreskin in place over the glans and also drawing it back over the glans (reversion) after the foreskin has been retracted (eversion).

AT WHAT AGE WILL THE FORESKIN FREELY RETRACT?

At birth, the foreskin is usually attached to the glans (head) of the penis, very much as a fingernail is attached to a finger.[8] By the end of puberty, the penis will usually have completed its development, and the foreskin will have separated from the glans.[9] Separation of the glans and foreskin occurs as a result of hormones secreted during childhood and puberty.[10] Erections, which naturally induce the foreskin to retract, also stimulate the separation process. This separation occurs in its own time.

It is very important to realize that there is no set age by which the foreskin and glans must be separated. Even if the glans and foreskin separate naturally in infancy, the lips of the foreskin can normally dilate only enough to allow the passage of urine. This ideal feature protects your young son's glans from premature exposure to the external environment.

The penis develops naturally throughout childhood. Eventually, the child will, on his own, make the wondrous discovery that his foreskin will retract. There is no reason for parents, physicians, or other caregivers to manipulate a child's penis. The only person to retract a child's foreskin should be the child himself, and only when he has discovered that his foreskin is ready to retract.

Parents should protect their child from doctors who try to retract his foreskin. Many doctors never learned about the normal development and care of the penis and are unaware that the foreskin should never be retracted by anyone, except its owner, and only when the penis has matured enough to make retraction free and easy.

WHY ISN'T THE FORESKIN USUALLY RETRACTABLE UNTIL THE TEENAGE YEARS?

There is no need for the foreskin to be retractable until puberty. Only then are humans biologically programmed to become sexually mature. In babies and young children, the natural attachment of the foreskin to the glans protects the immature glans from injury and dirt. The firmly attached foreskin provides a natural protective barrier for the urinary tract. This is especially important in infancy and during the diaper-wearing years. Of equal importance, the attachment of the foreskin to the glans *protects* and *preserves* the head of the penis, allowing it to complete its development.

IS IT NECESSARY FOR THE FORESKIN TO BE RETRACTABLE IN ADULTHOOD?

No. Many adults enjoy the comfort and security of a glans that is covered most or all of the time—even during erection. At this stage of life, the foreskin almost always has fully separated from the head. Full retraction is sometimes avoided if the lips of the foreskin (the preputial orifice) resist stretching wide enough to permit the passage of the glans. There is nothing wrong with this, even though many old-fashioned textbooks and many uninformed doctors (most of whom are circumcised) think that this is a problem called "phimosis."

Contrary to medical myth, a narrow preputial orifice does not make hygiene difficult. On the contrary: Important studies have found that the penis with a narrow foreskin opening is perfectly clean.[11] Urination through the foreskin actually helps keep the penis clean and fresh. It is a beautifully designed system that functions with perfect efficiency.

SPECIAL MOISTENERS AND EMOLLIENTS IN THE FORESKIN

All skin surfaces of the body require the constant moisturizing and soothing action of *sebum*—natural skin oil. Without it, the skin would dry out, crack, and bleed. To prevent this from occurring, the skin of the body is richly supplied with sebaceous glands. The natural secretion of skin oil gives the skin a healthy luster and enables it to do its job protecting the internal structures of the body from the external environment. Like skin, mucous membranes also require constant moistening. The mucous membranes of the eyes, for instance, are constantly bathed in moistening tears and other lubricating secretions from sebaceous glands in the inner eyelid. Similarly, the surfaces of the penis also require lubrication and moistening.

PREPUTIAL SEBUM (SMEGMA) AND ITS IMPORTANT ANTIBACTERIAL PROPERTIES

Preputial sebum, or *smegma*, is the creamy white emollient that can sometimes be found coating the inner lining of the foreskin.[12] It is a combination of secretions from many glands around the penis and urethra.[13]

Smegma is probably the most misunderstood, most unjustifiably maligned substance in nature. Smegma is clean rather than dirty. It is beneficial and necessary. It moisturizes the glans and keeps it smooth, soft, and supple. Its antibacterial and antiviral properties keep the penis clean and healthy. All normal male and female mammals produce smegma. Dr. Thomas J. Ritter underscored its importance when he commented, "The vertebrate animal kingdom would be depleted without smegma."[14]

Children produce very little smegma. During adolescence, the production of smegma markedly increases as the glands of the penis develop, perhaps in response to elevated testosterone levels. In adulthood, much less smegma is produced.

It is natural that smegma would be most abundant during adolescence and young adulthood, since this is the time when males are at their peak of sexual drive and when human males are biologically programmed to engage in mating. Smegma is most needed at this time to facilitate the smooth operation of the penis.

Apart from its lubricating function, smegma has antibacterial effects, most especially during infancy. Antibacterial substances are passed from mother to child during breast-feeding and are secreted in the baby's urine. Breast-fed babies receive substantial amounts of beneficial compounds called *oligosaccharides*.[15] When ingested, these compounds are secreted in the urine where they prevent certain types of bacteria from adhering to the urinary tract and the inner lining of the foreskin.

Animal experiments have found that special cells called *plasma cells* in the inner fold of the foreskin secrete a compound called *immunoglobulin*.[16] These secretions protect the penis against harmful bacteria. It is interesting to note that these antibacterial secretions increase in response to bacterial invasion.

SPECIALIZED NERVE RECEPTORS IN THE FORESKIN

The innervation of the foreskin is impressive.[17] Genitally intact males know from personal experience that the foreskin is one of the most sensitive parts of the body. Consequently, for over a century, some of the most respected names in medical science have turned their attention to this part of the body. Anatomists have transformed this inner knowledge into careful scientific observations about the complex innervation of the foreskin.

As the most richly innervated part of the penis, the foreskin has the largest number of nerve receptors, as well as the greatest variety of nerve receptors. These specialized nerve endings include Meissner's corpuscles,[18] free nerve endings, end bulbs of Krause,[19] corpuscles of Ruffini,[20] Pacinian corpuscles,[21] genital end bulbs,[22] genital bodies,[23] Merkel's disks, Golgi-Mazzoni corpuscles,[24] and Vater-Pacinian corpuscles.[25] These remarkable organs provide the foreskin with an amazing ability to detect the slightest sensations of touch, motion, temperature, and pressure. We are still unaware of all the facts about these fascinating structures. Future research may discover even more nerve receptors in the foreskin and help clarify what useful purposes they serve.

EROGENOUS ZONES OF THE FORESKIN

The foreskin is what's known as a *specific erogenous zone*.[26] This means that it is richly equipped with a high density and concentration of specialized and sophisticated nerve receptors that convey pleasure. The only other specific erogenous zones on the male body are the conjunctiva of the eye, lips, nipples, perianal skin, and the head of the penis. The presence of specialized erogenous nerve receptors makes this part of the body especially important.

The primary zones of erotogenous sensitivity are the frenulum, ridged mucosa, the preputial orifice, and the external fold of the foreskin. All of these zones are orgasmic triggers. Continuous and gentle stimulation of any one of these areas can elicit pleasure, orgasm, and ejaculation.

HOW THE GLANS COMPARES WITH THE FORESKIN

Most people are surprised to learn that the glans penis is one of the *least* sensitive parts of the entire body.[27] Obviously, this news may be worrying for circumcised males. The glans is insensitive to light touch, heat, cold, and even to pinpricks, as researchers at the Department of Pathology in the Health Sciences Centre at the University of Manitoba discovered.[28] The corona of the glans contains scattered free nerve endings, genital end bulbs, and Pacinian corpuscles, which transmit sensations of pain and deep pressure. The glans is nearly incapable of detecting light touch.

The nerve receptors of the corona are designed to be stimulated through the medium of the foreskin. Direct stimulation of the glans of the intact penis is most pleasant when the stimulus mimics the moist, massaging action of the foreskin.

The moving ring of pressure created by the lips of the foreskin and ridged mucosa stimulate the nerve receptors in the rim of the glans. While pleasurable stimulation of the frenulum and ridged mucosa is instantly perceived, sensation of the corona is slow and gradual. When fully stimulated, the erotic sensations felt in the corona are perceived as having a slow, warm, and rich quality. As nice as this is, it hardly compares to the erotic sensations generated by the foreskin. Circumcised males have been robbed of a normal body part. They have also been robbed of a normal level of sexual sensation. Just as a person whose lips were amputated could never really appreciate the sensations that lips can convey, so a circumcised male can never understand what his genitally intact friends experience. This helps explain why some circumcised males defend circumcision so vehemently. They have no idea what was taken from them and are psychologically unprepared to deal with their loss.

ISN'T THE FORESKIN A VESTIGIAL ORGAN
LIKE THE APPENDIX?

No. First of all, the appendix is hardly a vestigial organ. This myth was created back in the nineteenth century when medical science was too primitive to figure out the purpose of the appendix. Doctors back then were foolish enough to think that any organ whose function they were unable to understand was functionless and vestigial. Nowadays, we know the appendix to be an important part of the immune system, producing large quantities of lymphocytes and pumping them into the small intestine.

Similarly, the myth that the foreskin is a vestigial organ was invented by circumcisers as an additional justification for imposing mass circumcision on the American people. The foreskin cannot be vestigial. The results of a fascinating study conducted by Dr. Christopher Cold and Dr. Kenneth A. McGrath demonstrate that the human foreskin is an evolutionary advancement over the foreskins of other primates. The human foreskin is far more sophisticated and responsive, as their comparative anatomy studies prove. This is seen most clearly in the evolutionary increase in corpuscular innervation of the human foreskin and the simultaneous decrease in corpuscular receptors in the human glans relative to the innervation of the foreskin and glans of lower primates.[29] In other words, in monkeys and apes, the glans is more sensitive than the foreskin. In humans, this is reversed, so that the foreskin is more sensitive than the glans. If the foreskin were "vestigial," this advancement would never have taken place and the human foreskin would be either equally or less sensitive than the ape foreskin.

It is important to remember that there are no vestigial organs or body parts. Each and every part of the body serves a specific, important purpose. If the foreskin failed to serve a purpose, it would have disappeared millions of years ago. Drs. Cold and McGrath conclude that, over the last 65 million years, the foreskin has offered *reproductive advantages.* It must also be remembered that sexual selection has refined the external genitalia of every creature, including man. The human foreskin is the product of millions of years of evolutionary refinement, and, as such, the human foreskin represents the epitome of design perfection.

Chapter Two

● ● ●

The Functions of the Foreskin

The prepuce is primary, erogenous tissue necessary for normal sexual function. The complex interaction between the protopathic sensitivity of the corpuscular receptor-deficient glans penis and the corpuscular receptor-rich ridged band of the male prepuce is required for normal copulatory behavior.[1]

Christopher J. Cold, M.D., and John R. Taylor, M.D.

Now that you know what the foreskin is, you are probably wondering what it does. Most people are interested to learn that the foreskin has a great number of important protective, sensory, and sexual functions.

THE FORESKIN IN BABYHOOD

Babies are born perfect. Every part of your baby's body is there for a special purpose. Every part of your baby's body helps him grow, develop, learn, and experience our wondrous world. The foreskin is one of these special body parts. In fact, the foreskin is an important body part throughout the entire life of the male.

The foreskin adds more to the penis than just increased sexual functioning and pleasure. It keeps your baby's penis safe, warm, clean, and moist. It allows the baby's glans to complete its development normally. The glans is meant to be an internal organ, covered and protected from the outside world.

No attempt should be made to retract the foreskin before the penis has fully developed. Premature retraction causes the glans (the head) to become dry, hard, and scarred. The foreskin protects the glans from injury simply by covering it. The first person to retract the foreskin and expose the glans should be the child himself, and only when the child is ready to do so. It is best that parents avoid concerning themselves with this natural process. All by themselves, little boys will make the discovery that their foreskin can be retracted.

PROTECTION

Just as the eyelid protects the eye, the foreskin protects the glans, keeping its surface soft, moist, warm, and sensitive. It also maintains optimal warmth, pH balance, and cleanliness. The glans itself contains no sebaceous glands—glands that produce the moisturizing oil that our skin needs to stay healthy.[2] The foreskin produces the moisturizer that keeps the surface of the glans glistening, smooth, soft, and a deep healthy red or purple color.

The foreskin will protect the entire penis when accidents happen, such as contusions, abrasions, lacerations, and burns. The foreskin is the first layer—a double layer—of defense from injury to the rest of the penis.

SELF-CLEANSING FUNCTION

The intact penis is naturally clean. The common view of the penis or the foreskin as "dirty" is unscientific and irrational.

The penis, however, does provide an entry point into the body, and it is exposed to foreign microbes every day, especially during sexual intercourse. The immunological functions of the foreskin and the self-cleansing functions of the penis *protect* the body from harm.

Every time a genitally intact male urinates, the urine stream flushes out the urethra and foreskin of foreign microbes that may have strayed inside. In healthy individuals, urine is sterile and has a disinfectant quality. Researchers have demonstrated that the swirling action of urine as it rushes through the foreskin flushes it out effortlessly and naturally.[3] This function is especially efficient when the foreskin is long and the preputial orifice is narrow.

Though urine passes through the foreskin every day, the inner foreskin is remarkably free of urea—a by-product of liver metabolism that is secreted in the urine. Studies demonstrate that washings from the foreskin are rich in fructose, acid phosphatase, and mucin, but never urea. It appears that the secretions of seminal vesicles, prostate, and urethral mucous glands, collectively or individually, keep the foreskin clear and clean as well.[4] These self-cleansing functions of the penis are analogous to the self-cleansing functions of the eye, which similarly maintains its cleanliness through fluid washings (tears) and mucus secretion. Therefore, you never need to worry about the foreskin being "unclean."

SELF-PROTECTING FUNCTIONS

The urinary meatus (the opening of the glans through which urine and semen flow), is an entry point into the body. From infancy to adulthood, the foreskin ensures optimal protection of the glans and urinary meatus from contaminants of all kinds. During childhood, the foreskin is also usually firmly attached to the glans to prevent contaminants from invading the urethra. The neck of the foreskin places the vulnerable urinary meatus at a distance from the external environment and defends it against invading contaminants. The fusion of the foreskin and glans and the nonexpandability of the preputial orifice in the child's penis are therefore necessary for the health of the child. Even after the foreskin separates from the glans and becomes retractable, it continues throughout life to cover the glans and meatus in order to protect these delicate structures from dirt, contamination, abrasion, or bacterial invasion.

IMMUNOLOGICAL PROTECTION

The mucous membranes that line all body orifices are the body's first line of immunological defense. Glands in the foreskin produce antibacterial and antiviral proteins such as lysozyme.[5] Lysozyme is also found in tears and mother's milk. Specialized epithelial Langerhans cells, an immune system component, abound in the foreskin's outer surface.[6] Plasma cells in the foreskin's mucosal lining secrete immunoglobulins, antibodies that defend against infection.[7]

Rigorously controlled studies have also demonstrated that the foreskin plays a protective role in shielding the rest of the penis and thus the rest of the body from the contagion of common sexually transmitted diseases (STDs) encountered during sexual activity.[8] We will discuss this in more detail in Chapter 8.

In infancy, antibacterial substances, such as the simple sugars in breast milk, the oligosaccharides, are passed from mother to child during breast-feeding and are secreted in the baby's urine.[9] The penis retains these substances in the foreskin. University studies have shown that these substances protect against urinary tract infections, as well as infections of other parts of the body.[10] Babies excrete in their urine 300–500 milligrams of oligosaccharides a day. These compounds prevent virulent strains of *Escherichia coli* from adhering to the mucosal lining of the entire urinary tract, including the foreskin and glans.

Researchers conducting immunological experiments with the foreskins of bulls have found that plasma cells in the mucosal lining of the foreskin secrete immunoglobulin.[11] The researchers hypothesize that this provides immunity from bacteria and other germs. This may be true for humans as well.

Apocrine glands are important glands found in the skin. They are found in the foreskin and elsewhere on the body.[12] They secrete the important lysosomal enzymes cathepsin B, lysozyme, chymotrypsin, and neutrophil elastase.[13] All of these enzymes help protect the body from many kinds of bacteria. These enzymes are also found in tears and other bodily fluids. Human apocrine glands also produce cytokine, a nonantibody protein that generates an immune response on contact with specific antigens.[14] All these substances have immunological functions and protect the penis from viral and bacterial pathogens. This natural protective function has been destroyed in circumcised males.

ANTIBACTERIAL FUNCTION

To help fight harmful bacteria, the foreskin supports a rich flora of beneficial bacteria. Friendly bacteria exist in a symbiotic relationship with the body and are found on all body surfaces and throughout the gastrointestinal, genitourinary tract (the urinary system that runs from the kidneys, through the bladder, and out the penis), and the mouth. Friendly bacteria also thrive in the eyes. Without the presence of friendly bacteria, the human body would be vulnerable to attack from pathogenic bacteria.

The good bacteria that live in the inside of the foreskin are similar to the bacteria found in the mouth, nose, the female genitals, and the skin in general. It must be stressed that this good bacteria is both harmless and highly beneficial. Without these friendly bacteria, the urethra would become an easy entry point for germs and harmful strains of bacteria, which could cause disease.

COVERAGE DURING ERECTION

During erection, the penile shaft becomes thicker and longer. In some males, the penis can extend to twice its flaccid length. Sometimes, it can become even longer. The double-layered foreskin provides exactly the right amount of skin necessary to accommodate the expanded organ and to allow the penile skin to glide freely, smoothly, and pleasurably over the shaft and glans.

It is important to consider the fact that every penis is unique. By looking at an infant's penis, it is impossible to predict how big his penis will become when he is an adult. Heredity does play a role in determining the ultimate shape, size, and configuration of the penis, but it is still difficult to predict the adult size and shape of an infant's penis even if one looks at the penises of his father, brothers, and other male relatives.

What we can say with certainty is that your baby's penis will develop and mature according to his own unique genetic coding. Thus, the amount of foreskin he is born with is exactly the amount he will need for his penis to develop properly and experience comfortable, pleasurable erections throughout life. As a result, the idea that any amount of penile skin can be cut off without affecting the later function of the penis is false. In nature there is no surplus, only economy. Everything provided is required.

In the natural penis, as the shaft elongates during erection, the lips of the foreskin slowly expand. The glans begins slowly to protrude through the widening opening. Since the foreskin is soft, elastic, and pliable, it can easily and comfortably stretch to allow the passage of the glans. The stretching process elicits pleasurable sensations as the foreskin gently unrolls (everts) over the glans and shaft. Eventually, in most males, the glans can be fully exposed.

Some males, well endowed with a generous foreskin, have the glans fully covered even when the penis is fully erect. Most, however, if they choose, can manually roll the foreskin all the way back to expose the glans.

During full erection, the sensitive inner sleeve of the foreskin is turned inside out, exposing it. In this position it receives and transmits pleasurable sensations. The natural penis is a marvelously engineered organ for receiving and giving natural pleasure.

Needless to say, circumcision destroys all these functions and imposes a diminished, scarred, immobile, dowel-like penis that has permanently lost the ability to experience normal levels of sexual sensations. A circumcised male, or his partner, for that matter, can never know the intimacy of the normal penis and the ability of the foreskin to open and glide up and down the shaft. An entire dimension of sexuality has been lost to both the male and his sexual partner.

EROGENOUS SENSITIVITY

The foreskin is more sensitive than the fingertips or the lips of the mouth. It contains a richer variety and greater concentration of specialized nerve receptors than any other part of the penis.[15] These specialized nerve endings can discern motion, subtle changes in temperature, and fine gradations of texture.[16] This function enables genitally intact males to experience a superior dimension of sexual pleasure, compared to males who were circumcised. Intact males can be more tender, gentle, relaxed, and loving during sex because the slightest and subtlest gesture or motion evokes deeply satisfying sensations. Circumcised males have to work harder just to feel sensations. This is an unhealthy situation for both the male and his female partner.

SELF-STIMULATING SEXUAL FUNCTIONS

The intact penis has moving parts. The foreskin's double-layered sheath enables the penile shaft skin to glide back and forth over the penile shaft. The foreskin can usually be slipped all the way, or almost all the way, back to the base of the penis, and also slipped forward beyond the glans. This wide range of motion stimulates the orgasmic triggers in the foreskin, frenulum, and glans.

This is the natural way that the penis is erotically stimulated. The movement of the foreskin over the glans and the pressure of the glans pressing against the foreskin is pleasurable.

Sadly, males circumcised at birth can never imagine the pleasure of this natural sensation.

In the natural penis, the foreskin is the most important source of erotogenic, orgasm-inducing sensations. As we learned in the previous chapter, the foreskin contains a highly organized erotogenic sensory nerve-receptor system. It transmits special sexual sensations to the central nervous system and brain. The glans also has erotogenic sensory nerve receptors along its rim (the corona glandis), but far fewer than the foreskin. The massaging action of the foreskin against the glans produces sexual stimulation in both organs—something else that the circumcised male will never experience.

Some genitally intact males can even stimulate themselves to orgasm without touching their penis. They simply clench the groin muscles that help fill the penis with blood. Each voluntary contraction of the muscles forces more blood into the erectile tissues. This causes the shaft and glans to engorge even further and pushes the glans through the lips of the foreskin. Each dilation of the lips of the foreskin stimulates the specialized nerve receptors in the foreskin. In addition, the tension exerted on the foreskin stimulates the nerve receptors in the glans. The resulting sensation can lead to orgasm. A circumcised male would never be able to accomplish this natural feat.

THE FORESKIN ENHANCES FOREPLEASURE

Forepleasure is the pleasurable stimulation of the genitals with or without the intention of eliciting orgasm. Forepleasure takes place during foreplay. Forepleasure of the penis stimulates the brain to release beneficial and health-giving hormones into the bloodstream. These hormones improve overall bodily health, improve the emotional state, and can even reduce pain in any part of the body. Forepleasure, as the name implies, feels great.

Orgasm and ejaculation are usually the smallest part of sexual activity. They take only a few seconds and generally signal the end of sex interest. The period devoted to forepleasure is the greatest component of sexual activity and can continue as long as there is interest to do so. The intact penis is masterfully designed to give and receive forepleasure. Its many surfaces, structures, and moving parts lend themselves to pleasurable exploration. Unrolling the foreskin and exposing the glans is an intimate discovery that provides fascination and delight, since different parts of the penis respond to different kinds of pleasurable attentions. The exploration and discovery of these differences provide a lifetime of intimate enjoyment and satisfaction.

SEXUAL FUNCTIONS OF THE FORESKIN DURING INTERCOURSE

One of the foreskin's functions is to facilitate smooth, gentle, and slow movement between the two partners during intercourse. The foreskin enables the penis to slip in and out of the vagina nonabrasively inside its own slick sheath of self-lubricating, movable skin. The female is thus stimulated by moving pressure rather than by friction only, as when the male's foreskin is missing.

The foreskin fosters intimacy between the two partners by enveloping the glans and maintaining it as an internal organ. The sexual experience is enhanced when the foreskin slips back to allow the male's internal organ, the glans, to meet the female's internal organ, the cervix—a moment of supreme intimacy and beauty.

You may have heard circumcision promoters allege that the foreskin is "dangerously thin and delicate" and that it "rips and tears easily during sexual intercourse." This is unscientific nonsense and has no basis in anatomical fact. I am sorry to say that it is a deception calculated to provide false reassurance to anxious circumcised males and to frighten parents into letting their children be circumcised. The simple truth is that the foreskin is perfectly designed to function effortlessly and pleasurably during sexual activity. Its double-layered integument is strong, flexible, and resilient. The foreskin is a durable and vigorous organ that enhances and facilitates sexual intercourse. If it didn't, it would have atrophied millions of years ago.

SELF-LUBRICATING FUNCTION

Analogous to the eyelid, the foreskin protects and preserves the sensitivity of the glans by maintaining optimal levels of moisture, warmth, pH balance, and cleanliness. The glans is an internal organ. The glans itself contains no sebaceous glands and relies on the foreskin for production and distribution of sebum to maintain proper epithelial lubrication. Lubrication is naturally secreted by Cowper's glands in the urethra. This clear fluid begins to flow out of the meatus as the male becomes sexually aroused.

During intercourse, this natural lubricant assists the male in inserting the penis into the vagina. Because the fluid is sheltered under the foreskin of the erect penis, it is less likely to dry up. Instead, it keeps the penis well lubricated and prevents the vagina from drying out.

In the circumcised penis, the Cowper's gland fluid quickly evaporates. When the circumcised male inserts his dry penis into the vagina, it soon uses up all the female's natural lubricants, causing friction and pain for both partners. This can lead to small tears and painful bleeding in the organs of both partners. It comes as no surprise that in the United States today, where a large majority of sexually active adult males have been circumcised, painful vaginal dryness is the biggest complaint women have about sex. This is also the reason that there is such a large industry in the United States that manufactures artificial sexual lubricants. I doubt that there has ever been a study to determine the long-term effects of using these chemicals on such delicate organs.

Genitally intact males are free of the need for lubricants of any kind either for manual stimulation of the penis or for vaginal intercourse.

Many circumcised males must also resort to using these artificial factory-made lubricants to masturbate. Other circumcised males reach orgasm by friction of their hand over their externalized glans. They have been deprived of the gliding movement of the foreskin to stimulate themselves naturally. The penis is a different organ without a foreskin, and sexual function is altered when the foreskin has been amputated.

Many circumcised men will think they are normal because they are able to function sexually to their satisfaction, never realizing that their sexual functioning as an adult was changed forever by a medically unnecessary and extremely painful procedure done to them as an infant.

In my practice, I have examined little boys who have had so much foreskin removed that there is hardly any loose skin on their penis. The skin on their flaccid nonerect penis is taut. I wonder what will happen to a boy with such a radical circumcision when he gets an erection: Will he be able to have as much pleasure from his penis as he would have had if the circumciser had amputated less? This most unfortunate situation is all too common in the United States.

PRODUCTION, RETENTION, AND
DISPERSAL OF PHEROMONES

The sense of smell is one of the oldest, most precise, and most important senses in humans. Smells convey vital information to the brain. *Pheromones* are hormonal chemical messengers secreted by an individual and perceived by another individual of the same species. They create sexual arousal and attraction in the person perceiving the pheromone. These glands are found in the armpits, breasts, and in the genital area. The penis itself is a specific site for these glands. Pheromones may well be secreted by the apocrine glands in the foreskin. These glands are present at birth, but during puberty they develop in the presence of testosterone.

Although pheromones themselves are odorless, they are released by the foreskin into the air where they are perceived by the *vomeronasal organ,* a small tubular structure in the mucosa of the nasal septum. This organ is a component of the accessory olfactory system. The olfactory area of the cerebral cortex is closely associated with the limbic system, the part of the brain that organizes emotional responses, mood, memory, and sexual arousal. Although most complex smells and their emotional associations are learned, the identification of pheromones is hardwired into the brain. The automatic sexual arousal elicited by the perception of pheromones is as certain as the automatic pleasure reflex elicited by a caress.

The perception of any scent associated with pheromones varies from individual to individual and depends largely on bacteria. The bacteria itself may be needed to chemically interact with the pheromones to make them active.[17] Diet, bathing habits, and general health also affect the quality of these scents. The predominant odor associated with male pheromones is musk. Nearly all human cultures esteem the rich, earthy, musky, pheromone-rich scent produced by the glands in the foreskin. Perfume makers obtain musk from the foreskin glands of the musk deer. The nonhuman pheromones contained in this musk are unable to elicit sexual arousal in humans, but the fragrance of the musk itself may, by association, elicit a pleasant response in humans that evokes a sympathetic erotic arousal.[18] This is, at least, the effect that the perfume industry hopes to create.

Chapter Three

•••

What Happens to a Baby During a Circumcision?

In the eyes of the physician, this barbaric tradition of unnecessary surgery is a thing of the past and should take its place in history books as one of the many traditions that a humane civilization has outgrown.[1]

Carl Otten, M.D.

A newborn baby boy is amazing! He can see, hear, smell, taste, think, and feel. He can and does experience pain and pleasure. These abilities have been known to mothers since the dawn of man. Yet, these obvious characteristics of human behavior have seldom been acknowledged by surgeons and psychologists. It was only in the last quarter of the twentieth century that doctors were willing to admit that babies could feel pain. Of course, it now seems obvious to any observer who hears an agonizing cry that a baby can indeed feel pain.

It is my sad duty to inform you that there is no scientific debate that circumcising the penis is extremely traumatizing and stressful for baby boys. This fact has been extensively documented in the medical literature. Why, then, are some people—including doctors who perform the surgery—reluctant to accept this truth?

My feeling is that, on a day-to-day basis, we choose to ignore things that disturb us. The trauma of circumcision is so gruesome and upsetting that most people prefer to minimize, ignore, or deny it. The fact that the sex organs are involved, the frightening-looking surgical instruments, the blood, the gore, and the agonizing, frenzied screaming of the baby are all too much for any normal, sane, and compassionate individual to handle without resorting to unfounded beliefs, myths, and superstitions. Most surgeons who perform circumcision have suppressed their humanity and sense of compassion. They have desensitized themselves as a way of coping with a brutal reality that they feel powerless to change. People accept this situation because they have been misled into thinking that it is essential for their survival to have this brutal procedure performed on themselves, or, even worse, on their children.

Few people want accurate and complete information on circumcision because it is so horrifying, and they fear that they would be unable to handle it. It is easier to block it out. Dealing with the facts is too painful. Doctors must be trained and conditioned to desensitize themselves to stomach-turning and repulsive scenes because there is no other way that they could help injured people.

Just stop for a moment, though, and think: If the actual procedure of circumcision is too horrifying and disturbing for adults to think about, what about the babies forced to experience it? As compassionate and intelligent human beings, we owe it to our children to face the facts and act in a responsible manner. Ignoring the facts will hardly make them go away. Our children have no one else to defend them. Parents who want to do the right thing have a moral duty to protect their children from pain and trauma, and your best weapon with which to defend your children is *the truth.*

Most parents are unaware of what is actually done to a baby when he is circumcised. This is to be expected because the surgery excludes parents and occurs behind closed doors and in special soundproof circumcision chambers that are hidden deep inside U.S. hospitals. Parents are usually not permitted to watch. Parents are also never told what actually occurs in these circumcision chambers. If they were told what really happens during the surgery, it is doubtful that any parents would allow it to happen to their precious new baby.

Some parents who have witnessed a circumcision or who have seen a videotape of one have been so shocked that they have vowed that they will protect their children from this painful and traumatic experience. As Melissa Morrison explained, seven months after watching the circumcision of her baby son:

> *It's absolutely horrible. I didn't know how horrific it was going to be. It was the most gruesome thing I have ever seen in my life. I told the doctor as soon as he was done, if I had a gun I would have killed him.*[2]

Another mother who witnessed her son being circumcised confessed that:

> *The screams of my baby remain embedded in my bones and haunt my mind.*[3]

This chapter contains very graphic information that some readers will find disturbing. As hard as it will be for you to read, it is even harder for a baby to endure. I think that you owe it to yourself and to your child to inform yourself of every aspect of the circumcision surgery. See a video of a circumcision. Read the following descriptions. Hold your precious and perfect baby in your arms or at your breast before you make any decision.

PRELIMINARY STAGES

The pain caused by circumcision may be so severe that many babies frequently vomit during the operation. Occasionally, the child will choke and suffocate on his own vomit.[4] To avoid this, some hospitals deny the newborn baby any food for at least two hours before the surgery. In the first week of life, babies need to nurse very frequently. Denying babies food when they need it puts them at risk for hypoglycemia and jaundice. Any sensible person instinctively understands that it is wrong to deny newborn babies food for any period of time, except, perhaps, under the most extraordinary life-or-death medical emergencies. Routine circumcision hardly qualifies as a surgery performed for emergency reasons. You may be interested to know that researchers have never performed any studies to document the consequences of starving newborns in this manner, even though it is standard practice in many hospitals.

Once the baby has been "prepared" like this, he is taken into the circumcision chamber where the cutting will occur. As you will recall from earlier chapters, a baby's foreskin and glans are attached to each other, very much the way the eyelids of a newborn kitten are sealed closed. The foreskin and glans may remain attached to each other until after puberty. Therefore, before the foreskin can be amputated, it must first be torn from the glans.

The very fact that the foreskin must be torn from the glans means that it is supposed to be attached. The baby's foreskin is hardly an easily removable body part. It is attached to the glans for at least four important reasons:

1. The baby's penis is still undergoing development.
2. The glans does not need to be exposed during babyhood.
3. The natural attachment of the foreskin to the glans protects the immature glans from injury and dirt.
4. The firmly attached foreskin provides a natural protective barrier for the urinary tract. This is especially important in infancy.

Therefore, working against nature, the circumciser straps the baby's arms and legs down spread-eagle to a restraining board.[5] The circumciser then rubs the baby's penis with a disinfectant. This step may be performed by a nurse or assistant.

Because penile tissue is erectile tissue, it may respond to this stimulation by becoming erect. Next, the circumciser clamps the tissue at the edge of the foreskin opening at two places with clamps called *hemostats* that tightly grip the tissue. Then the circumciser will force a long, blunt probe or another hemostat between the foreskin and the glans. He forces the probe around the circumference of the glans, tearing the foreskin away from the glans. In my mind, I can still hear babies' cries and screams of agony as I write this.

Studies show that this tearing procedure is one of the most traumatically painful stages of the surgery.[6] Imagine having an instrument forced all the way under your fingernail and then moved back and forth before tearing off the nail. This is the level of unbearable pain that a baby experiences at this stage of the surgery. What follows, however, is far worse. This procedure may cause delicate pieces of tissue to be ripped out of the glans—like the flesh of an orange sometimes adheres to the peel—leaving a pitted, pockmarked surface.

Next, the circumciser inserts one blade of the long, scissors-like *mosquito clamp* into the foreskin above the glans and clamps it shut. This crushes the foreskin along a single line from the opening of the foreskin to the rim of the glans (the coronal sulcus). This is supposed to prevent bleeding, but it frequently fails in this respect. After a few minutes, the circumciser releases the clamp and cuts along the line of crushed tissue with scissors. This creates a dorsal incision from the opening of the foreskin to the rim of the glans, and frequently beyond this point down the shaft of the penis. The circumciser now peels back the divided layers of the foreskin to expose the raw and bleeding glans, which was never intended to be exposed until it had completed its development during puberty.

THE AMPUTATION OF THE FORESKIN

Once the stages above have been completed, the damaged foreskin is amputated. There are a variety of methods used in American hospitals today to cut off the foreskin. One common feature of each of these methods is that they destroy the foreskin, but they also necessarily sever the frenulum—the band of highly sensitive and elastic tissue that tethers the foreskin to the bottom of the glans, just under the urinary opening of the glans (meatus). Under the misguided impression that they must destroy as much mucous membrane as possible, circumcisers have actually been trained to take a scalpel and carve out whatever remains of the frenulum. As a result, one of the most sensitive areas of the penis is permanently anesthetized. One wonders how a man could even reach orgasm with a penis that has been permanently numbed like this. This may be responsible for the high incidence of sexual dysfunction in circumcised American males.

Here are some of the most common methods of circumcision in use today.

Gomco Clamp

The most common instrument for amputating the foreskin is the Gomco clamp. It was invented in 1934 by Aaron Goldstein and Hiram S. Yellen.[7] Gomco is an acronym for the *Gold*stein *M*anufacturing *Co*mpany, which later changed its name to the Gomco Surgical Manufacturing Corporation of Buffalo, New York. This steel device is widely used today to crush the baby's foreskin prior to its amputation. It also mashes the crushed and wounded skin edges together. This device produces more pain and trauma than any other foreskin amputation procedure. Circumcision with the Gomco clamp usually takes between sixteen and thirty-six minutes.[8] It is a shockingly inhumane procedure, especially when used without any anesthesia, as is most often the case.

The circumciser places the removable metal bell of the clamp device over the glans penis. He stretches the two halves of the split foreskin back into place over the bell and pierces the foreskin with safety pins to hold the two edges of the divided foreskin over the bell. The circumciser pushes the penis with the bell over the glans through a hole in the bottom of the Gomco clamp device and snaps the bell handle onto the lever of the clamp. The bottom diameter of the bell is larger than the diameter of the hole on the clamp, and the foreskin becomes trapped between the edges of the hole and the bottom edge of the bell. The circumciser turns a thumbscrew on the clamp, pulling the base of the bell tight against the metal hole, and crushing the foreskin around its circumference.

The clamp is supposed to be held in this position for several minutes until the arteries and veins of the foreskin are thoroughly crushed, supposedly to prevent bleeding or hemorrhage. Next, the circumciser takes a scalpel and cuts through the two folds of the crushed foreskin until the scalpel meets the metal of the bell, then runs the scalpel along the base of the hole and amputates all the visible skin. The circumciser holds the clamp in position for another five minutes to reduce bleeding after it is removed. The circumciser loosens the thumbscrew and removes the remainder of the penis from the clamp. The crushing and clotting cause the stump of the penile skin system to stick to the metal bell, so the circumciser must peel the skin from the bell to remove the bell from the glans penis.

The circumciser has created two large circular wounds; that of the amputated inner fold of the foreskin and that of the outer surface of the foreskin. The Gomco clamp crushes the edges of the wound together and only rarely will the circumciser suture the edges. Eventually, the two raw edges will adhere and scar over. The large scar that results from circumcision is the point where the two edges have been spliced together. Scarring takes a week or so to form.

The Gomco clamp has crippled countless boys. Using the Gomco clamp, circumcisers have amputated the foreskin, along with the rest of the skin of the penis.[9] The bell of the device can stick to the glans, obliging the circumciser to peel the bell off the penile stump, and in so doing, ripping open the shaft of the penis.[10] This is an exceptionally brutal way of treating babies. These clamps have been used on babies for almost seventy years without undergoing any safety improvements.

Plastibell

The plastic bell (Plastibell) method proceeds like the Gomco clamp method, but the bell inserted into the penis is made of molded plastic rather than metal. Instead of a clamp, a thin waxed string is tied so tightly around the foreskin over the bell as to cut off all circulation to the end of the penis. Like having a finger slammed in a door and kept there until it falls off the hand, the circumciser forces the baby to wear this penile strangulation device for a week or so until the end of the penis turns black, dies, and falls off, taking the plastic bell with it.

The Plastibell method is associated with many serious and tragic complications.[11] Among the many complications, the plastic ring may fail to fall off and instead become embedded in the penis, causing permanent deformity of the glans.[12] It will then have to be surgically removed. The Plastibell ring may also strangle the remnant penis, cutting off circulation, and resulting in infection, urinary retention, total denudation of the penis,[13] and gangrene.[14]

The plastic ring technique is also associated with life-threatening infections.[15] One frightening danger from Plastibell circumcision is necrotizing fasciitis, a rapidly spreading bacterial infection producing swelling, gangrene, and liquefaction of the remaining penis.[16] Even when no serious complications ensue, the Plastibell results in an especially prominent and darkly pigmented circumcision scar.

Electrocautery Gun

The electrocautery gun burns off the foreskin with a high-voltage current while the child is fully awake and unanesthetized. This method is popular with circumcisers despite the great danger it poses. In "minor" accidents, the electric gun can burn off all the skin of the penis.[17] In the most tragic instances, the electric current can broil the penis alive, causing it to drop off in a day or so. Most of the American baby boys who have been accidentally penectomized have lost their penises because the circumciser used an electrocautery gun on the child. The electrocautery gun should never be used with the Gomco clamp. I am saddened that so many circumcisers ignore this basic safety standard, preferring to impress themselves with their high-tech gadgets.

Many American boys, penectomized in this way, have been subjected to sex change operations to turn them into girls.[18] Needless to say, these unfortunate boys never asked to be circumcised in the first place. In the famous and tragic case of David Reimer, later known as John/Joan, the penis was burned off during a circumcision with an electrocautery gun.[19] On doctor's orders, this poor boy was subsequently subjected to a sex change operation and raised as a girl. As a teenager, when he discovered that he had been born a boy, he sued the doctors who did this to him and began the long process of restoring his life. I know that you will agree with me that no child should ever be forced to endure what this brave man has suffered.

Mogen Clamp

The Mogen clamp is another common circumcision device. After the circumciser tears the foreskin from the glans, he pulls the foreskin tightly away from the rest of the penis with small scissorslike clamps and places the open metal jaws of the Mogen clamp over the stretched foreskin. The circumciser closes and tightens the jaws with a lever. This crushes the foreskin between the two heavy metal blades of the clamp. With a scalpel, the circumciser slices off the protruding penile skin trapped in the jaws and keeps the jaws closed for a few minutes to make sure that all the blood vessels are crushed and have begun to clot. Then, the circumciser slowly opens the jaws of the clamp and removes it. The clamp has crushed the stump of the foreskin shut, trapping the glans inside. The circumciser places his fingers at the base of the penis and pulls the penile skin downward until the clotted seal breaks. The circumciser then takes up the blunt probe, sticks it into the wound, runs it along the glans, and tears apart any remaining attachment of the foreskin and glans.

After circumcision with the Mogen clamp, the stump of the foreskin has an asymmetrical, dog-eared appearance, as if it had been cut with pinking shears. There have recently been a large number of reports of tragic accidents involving the Mogen clamp. A number of boys have had their entire foreskin and glans penis amputated after they both were caught in the blades of the clamp.[20]

While I was writing this chapter, a mother called me from Texas with a very sad story. Her beautiful newborn son had been circumcised with a Mogen clamp on his second day of life. Horrifyingly, in addition to cutting off his precious foreskin, the circumciser caught half of the baby's glans in the Mogen clamp and sliced both structures off.

The baby required immediate reconstructive surgery. Under general anesthesia the severed glans was sewn back on, but leaving a large, angry scar where the glans had been amputated. That poor child must now endure life with two large scars on his penis—the circumcision scar on the shaft and the circumcision scar on the damaged glans. The boy's mother wanted advice on how to care for his damaged penis. All the doctors told her was that if the boy could urinate, he would be okay. They neglected to tell her about the inevitable physical, sexual, and emotional trauma this lad will unfairly have to endure for the rest of his life.

Sheldon Crushing Clamp

The Sheldon clamp resembles a large spring-hinged wood clamp. To perform the amputation, the circumciser first forces a blunt probe into the foreskin's opening and rips the foreskin away from the glans. He then pulls the foreskin into the open jaws of the device, clamps it shut, and locks it in place. Instead of cutting, the clamp *crushes* the foreskin in half. The circumciser then takes a knife and excises the foreskin and any other part of the penis that has been pulled into the clamp.

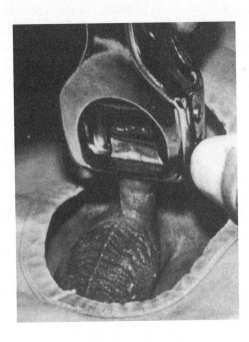

A baby's penis being circumcised by a Sheldon clamp

Photo courtesy of John A. Erickson.

The potential for accidents with the Sheldon clamp are high. *The Journal of Urology* recently reported a case of an American baby whose normal and healthy foreskin and glans were destroyed with this clamp.[21] The child is now a sexual cripple because of someone else's irrational compulsion to cut his sex organ. This is just one report. There are many other reports of similar accidents in the medical literature, while even more cases are covered up.

PAIN OF CIRCUMCISION

The pain that a baby experiences during circumcision is worse than anything the average person is likely to experience in a lifetime. Sadly, there is nothing that can be done to eliminate this pain entirely. Studies show that anesthesia helps reduce pain to some extent, but it is powerless to make circumcision pain free.

The pain of circumcision can have serious complications. It is so severe that many babies stop breathing, vomit, and defecate in their agony. One recent study on the pain of circumcision was stopped after several infants, circumcised without anesthesia, experienced life-threatening breathing difficulties that included choking and apnea.[22] The shock of circumcision results in hysterical screaming, crying, and can produce dangerous complications, including rupture of the heart,[23] lungs,[24] and stomach.[25]

Some babies are so severely traumatized by the experience that they fall into a semicomatose state. Some circumcisers still pretend that these babies are just falling asleep! Nothing could be further from the truth. No one falls asleep when his sex organs are being cut with a knife. Because he is tied down, a baby has no way to escape, no matter how much he thrashes. Going into a comalike state is one way for the baby to distance himself from his agony, but it has dangerous consequences for the brain, as you will read below.

When I was in medical school, I was taught to perform neonatal circumcisions without any anesthesia simply because it was commonly believed that the newborn was incapable of experiencing pain, and, even if he did, he would be unable to remember it. I accepted this because I had never heard of anyone remembering the trauma of being circumcised. Ethically, of course, we do not have the right to hurt another human being even if he won't remember the pain later.

It is unnecessary to be a university professor to understand that babies feel pain and are traumatized by circumcision. Just witness one—if you dare—and you will be convinced. You hardly need data collected by scientists to realize what those agonizing cries mean. You are a human being, capable of those same feelings. You know that even though the actual memory of the event may be lost, the trauma probably remains forever.

Many circumcisers still repeat the ludicrous myth that babies are unable to experience pain, even though they hear the screams of the babies. Many dismiss the evidence of their senses, and simply accuse the baby of being "fussy." It saddens me that members of my own profession could be so wrong, insensitive, and arrogant.

A mountain of objective scientific studies has irrefutably proved that babies do feel pain.[26] They feel it very acutely. In fact, it has now been conclusively established that babies feel pain more sharply than adults![27] Any mother who accidentally pokes her baby with a safety pin while changing diapers knows very well how sensitive babies are to pain. If a tiny pinprick can raise such a rush of pain and panic in a baby, imagine the baby's reaction to having a steel clamp crush the end of his penis or to having a scalpel slice it open.

Pain is serious. It is hardly something to be dismissed, laughed at, or ignored. Pain is hardly good for the soul, and it cannot "toughen" little boys. In fact, it has just the opposite effect. The severe pain of circumcision makes boys *less* able to tolerate even average levels of pain. A team of top-notch medical researchers working at the University of Toronto have proved in a series of studies that the pain of circumcision is so severe that it permanently damages the pain centers of the brain. Baby boys who have been circumcised suffer from an abnormally and artificially lowered pain threshold than genitally intact boys or baby girls. They react more strongly, violently, and hysterically to mildly painful experiences, such as vaccination injections.[28] Development neuropsychologist Dr. James Prescott suggests that circumcision can cause deeper and more disturbing levels of neurological damage, as well.[29] We must ask ourselves: What dangerous and dark message is being sent to the mind when the organ designed for experiencing pleasure becomes the source of unbearable pain? Dr. Prescott writes:

> *It is this writer's conviction that the extraordinary pain and trauma experienced through genital mutilations— an organ and brain system that is designed for the experience of sexual pleasure and the expression of sexual love—has permanently altered normative brain development for the normal expression of sexual pleasure and love. It is proposed that this genital pain has long-term developmental consequences for the ability of such individuals to differentiate pain from pleasure in love relationships and to develop intimate sexual relationships.*
>
> *It is not without psychobiological consequence that the brain system, which is designed for the experience of pleasure and the expression of sexual love, is first encoded with extraordinary and excruciating pain. In such individuals, all subsequent acts or experiences of genital pleasure are experienced upon a background of genital pain that is now deeply buried in the subconscious unconscious brain.*[30]

Pain is never a temporary experience. It persists even after the knife stops cutting. One powerful study performed at the University of Rochester School of Medicine documented the disturbing fact that babies still experience severe pain at least twenty-four hours after the circumcision surgery.[31] This study was able to measure pain for only twenty-four hours because most of the babies in the study were discharged from the hospital during this time. The excruciating pain undoubtedly lasts much longer.

Anyone who has had surgery knows that severe pain can last for weeks. Patients must usually take massive doses of powerful painkillers for a week or more. Tragically, babies are still being denied postoperative pain relief. Hospital routines are slow to adjust to scientific advances. Just as many hospital administrators still push circumcision, they also choose to ignore the overwhelming evidence that now exists on the pain of circumcision and refuse to require all circumcisers to use anesthesia.

The throbbing pain of the circumcision amputation wound is aggravated every time the baby urinates. Babies have no choice but to urinate into the raw circumcision wound. The hot acidic urine burns the raw flesh, inflicting even more genital pain. Nurses who work in maternity wards have told me that they can always tell which babies in the nursery have been circumcised. These poor babies act strangely and seem withdrawn. They also scream hysterically when they urinate in their diapers.

I strongly advise parents to avoid being misled into believing that wine on a pacifier or dripped into the baby's mouth through a bottle provides anesthesia or analgesia. The baby may become intoxicated, but this is dangerous and unhelpful itself. Some circumcisers wrongly claim that this method is useful. This is a falsehood. Also, you would be wise to resist the temptation to believe that sugar water (glucose) provides anesthesia or analgesia. Sugar may stimulate the opioid receptors in the brain, but this is hardly going to block the excruciating pain of circumcision. If a circumciser ever tries to talk you into letting him give your child a sugar solution while he cuts your child's penis, ask him if he would willingly substitute a bottle of cola for anesthesia before allowing a surgeon to cut *his* penis.

Even though the American Academy of Pediatrics now urges

circumcisers to use local anesthesia,[32] circumcisers almost universally ignore these recommendations.[33] They also ignore the fact that the American Academy of Pediatrics actually recommends protecting babies from circumcision in the first place. Many circumcisers are unwilling to change their habits or learn new techniques. Many have chosen to ignore the evidence that they are inflicting major harm on babies. Many just don't care. Consequently, most babies who are circumcised in U.S. hospitals today are denied any form of pain relief during and after the surgery. General anesthesia is extremely dangerous for babies and local anesthesia is largely ineffective, but does this mean that pain relief should be dismissed as unimportant? Hospital spokesmen complain that the death and complication rate from local anesthesia itself is a disincentive for using it. It is true that anesthesia has resulted in tragic injuries and deaths. What then are caring parents supposed to do? It is clear to me that the only moral way of protecting babies from pain, injury, and stress disorders is to protect them from circumcision.

ADDITIONAL DANGERS OF CIRCUMCISION

Another negative effect that circumcision has on the brain is the creation of abnormal sleep patterns. This effect is characterized by a decrease of REM (rapid eye movement) sleep, where the arousal continuum is at a low point, where thresholds to sensory stimulation are high, and where motor activity is low.[34] Normally, infants begin their sleep cycle with REM sleep, but after enduring the stress of being circumcised, infants experience prolonged non-REM sleep. This is abnormal, and it may have life-long negative consequences that science has failed to investigate.

Studies conducted at the Institute of Child Development at the University of Minnesota,[35] the Albert Einstein College of

Medicine,[36] and the University of Colorado School of Medicine[37] reveal that circumcised infants suffer from a detrimental shift in sleep pattern, staying awake for longer periods of time than they did before the surgery. Even when they are able to sleep, the amount of shallow sleep increases, and the crucial periods of deep sleep decrease. In order to try to calm themselves and ease the pain emanating from the surgical wound, circumcised babies suck harder, faster, and more vigorously at their bottles, making them less available to their environment, and less able to interact with their mothers.[38]

Independent studies conducted at Washington University School of Medicine,[39] the University of California at San Diego School of Medicine,[40] and the University of Rochester School of Medicine[41] have confirmed that circumcision can also lead to a disruption of breast-feeding and an impairment of infant-maternal attachment.[42] In a study at the Washington University School of Medicine, most babies were unable to nurse right after they were circumcised, and those who did nurse refused to look into their mothers' eyes.[43]

The fact that circumcision causes severe short-term sleep problems is proven beyond a shadow of a doubt. One may ask, however, whether these problems could extend into the long term. One highly suggestive study, conducted at Northwestern University Medical School in Chicago and published in 1984 provides tantalizing clues to this question. The study found that among four- to eight-month-old infants from middle-class American families, the problem of night waking was significantly greater among infant boys than among infant girls. Now, we must remember that this study was conducted at the height of the campaign for mass routine circumcision. Therefore, we can safely assume that the vast majority of the male babies in this study had been subjected to circumcision. It is important to note that these boys were free of any other sleep problems, such as snoring or mouth breathing, that could account for the difference. Likewise, the reported sleep problems were unrelated to the method of feeding.[44] Other studies have found similar results.[45] We owe it to ourselves and to our precious children to consider the possibility that circumcision is to blame for the increase in long-term sleep disorders among the male babies in this study.

After reading this chapter, you are probably shocked. You may be angry that doctors routinely withhold these facts from parents. These disturbing facts may have been withheld from you when you were unfairly put in the position of having to decide about the circumcision of your own children without adequate knowledge. After reading this book, you will probably know more about circumcision than your doctor.

There is a reason for this, but it is hardly a justification. You see, most male physicians in the United States are circumcised. They were born during the mass circumcision campaigns of the Cold War era. They are unaware of the many untoward effects of circumcision, since, being circumcised at birth, they are unable to compare their present state with how they might have experienced life had they been allowed to remain genitally intact. In medical school, almost none were ever taught anything useful or accurate about circumcision. Since many circumcised doctors have forced themselves to believe their bodies are "normal" despite having lost a significant portion of their penis, they naively reason that everyone who has been circumcised is also "normal." Most doctors have conveniently chosen to shield their egos and to believe that circumcision is a stress-free surgery without any negative consequences. Nothing could be further from the truth, as the medical literature proves.

The good news is that we really do have the power to protect our children from these distressing experiences. Circumcision is unnecessary. You can protect your baby from circumcision and all of its accompanying stresses, traumas, terrors, surgical risks, and lifelong disadvantages. Most parents who see what is done to a baby when he is circumcised and how he reacts choose to protect their baby from circumcision. Before you allow a circumciser to touch your child, I urge you to watch a videotape of a circumcision. You will be grateful that you learned the truth before submitting your precious baby to this distressing experience. Informative and sensitively produced videos, such as the *NOCIRC Circumcision Video,* or *Whose Body, Whose Rights?*, or *Circumcision? Intact Facts* can be ordered from the National Organization of Circumcision Information Resource Centers (NOCIRC). See Appendices B and C for contact details.

Chapter Four

• ● •

Proven Complications and Risks of Circumcision

The risks of newborn circumcision are an underreported and ignored factor in this argument. Most often a poor surgical result is
not recognized until years after the event.[1]

James L. Snyder, M.D.
Past President of the Virginia Urologic Society

Is there any normal adult male who would voluntarily submit
to the surgical reduction of the size of his penis? Yet, routine
newborn circumcision *is* penile reduction surgery, and, like all
surgery, it carries many serious risks, even when performed with
the skill of the most able surgeon. In fact, according to the medical literature, the majority of the most horrifying and tragic
complications have occurred at the hands of skilled surgeons.
Sadly, newborn circumcision is often the start of a long and
tragic medical history.

There is no trustworthy data on the true rate of circumcision complications reported in the medical literature, and, I am
sorry to say, even doctors are ignorant of this information. Be-

lieve it or not, hospitals are conveniently free of any obligation to report circumcision accidents. The best we can do is estimate the rate of complication using data and case reports that are occasionally published in medical journals. Additionally, circumcisers feel that they are free of any obligation to report to medical journals the cases where they cripple, maim, castrate, or kill a child. Some blame circumcision disasters on other things, such as infections, without admitting that the circumcision wound they inflicted provided an entry point for the infection. Many of the most horrific circumcision accidents actually have been reported in newspapers and magazines. Medical journals seem to steer clear of reporting accounts of doctor-caused circumcision harm.

It is best for parents to realize that it is *impossible* to predict which babies will experience a circumcision disaster. Because of the poor defenses newborn infants have against blood loss, infection, or severe injury, it is best to be conservative about offering or inflicting surgery at this age, especially in cases where the indications for surgery are "tenuous" at best. It is one thing to suffer a surgical accident while being treated for a life-threatening disease or injury; it is quite another thing to suffer a life-threatening surgical accident for an unnecessary surgery on a healthy body part. How would parents ever be able to explain to their child when he grew up that half—or even all!—of his penis was destroyed in an operation that he was forced to undergo just because his circumcised father insisted that the baby's penis "match" his?

Because the penis is involved, the potential is high for these risks to be horrifying and tragic. While an operation on the leg that results in amputation is devastating, the loss of the penis is even more so. In the hierarchy of body parts, the penis ranks among the most important in human psychology. A boy whose penis has been horribly mutilated or destroyed during circumcision is more likely to suffer a lifetime of severe psychological problems than a boy whose leg was damaged or accidentally amputated in a leg operation.

One study estimates that a realistic complication rate for newborn circumcision ranges from 2 to 10 percent.[2] To the many circumcised men who become aware of the function and value of the prepuce, the very fact that this sensory organ was destroyed is *itself* a complication of circumcision. As far as they are concerned, the actual complication rate is 100 percent. For males fortunate enough to survive the surgery without immediate complications, there is a growing awareness today of the long-term consequences of neonatal circumcision. These are only now beginning to be documented.

Circumcisers have led many parents to believe that circumcision is a safe operation. They have withheld from parents the documented fact that at least one out of every five hundred circumcisions in the United States results in a serious surgical accident.[3] Additionally, according to Dr. Christopher Fletcher of St. Vincent Hospital in Santa Fe, New Mexico, between 5 and 15 percent of circumcisions in the United States result in serious surgical mishaps requiring *reconstructive surgery.*[4] The medical literature is filled with articles documenting the many dangers of circumcision.[5]

One difficulty in determining the true rate of complication is that there is no set definition of what constitutes a complication. When the long-term complication of *meatal stenosis* (pathological closing of the urinary opening) is factored in, the rate rises dramatically. On this basis, one study concluded that complications occurred at an alarming rate of 55 percent.[6]

COMMON CIRCUMCISION DISASTERS

The following is a summary of the most common complications of circumcision. They are serious. Most are life-threatening. It is impossible for a circumciser to honestly guarantee that they won't occur. Yet, they are *all* entirely avoidable if parents protect their children from circumcision.

Bleeding

Bleeding, also known as hemorrhage, is a complication inherent in any surgical procedure. Bleeding is more than just a few drops of blood. It means dangerous and nearly uncontrollable blood loss as a result of severed arteries. American babies have bled to death from circumcision. Sometimes it is hard to tell that the baby is hemorrhaging because the blood can unnoticeably be absorbed by diapers. The reported incidence of bleeding after circumcision can vary from 0.1 to 35 percent.[7] Excessive bleeding can require a blood transfusion, but, as any doctor will tell you, blood transfusions carry the risk of infecting your baby with HIV and other blood-borne disease organisms.

In a medical journal report, Dr. John Van Duyn reported a typical case of severe bleeding that warrants consideration:

> *There is also a distinct danger from hemorrhage, especially if the baby is placed in the prone position and supervision is minimal. In a near fatality from this cause, of which I have firsthand knowledge, a ligature had apparently been rubbed off from one of the arteries near the frenum and a growing puddle of blood beneath the baby was not discovered for a considerable time.*[8]

A few years ago, I was called to see a baby on a Saturday evening after sundown. The baby had been circumcised that morning in a religious rite by a nonphysician circumciser. When the parents arrived at my office, I was horrified to see that the poor little baby's diaper was completely soaked with blood. The parents had been afraid to bother me because it was a Saturday and, crucially, because the circumciser had convinced them that the bleeding would stop if they would just wait. As it turns out, they almost waited too long. The baby had hemorrhagic disease of the newborn and would have bled to death if the parents had waited a moment longer. I was able to save this baby's life. Many babies are less lucky.

Infection

Serious, life-threatening infections may occur following circumcision. Studies have found that the rate of serious postcircumcision infection can be as high as 10 percent.[9] Virulent infectious germs can easily enter the circumcision wound because it is so large. Unfortunately, due to overuse of antibiotics and antiseptic cleansers, many dangerous strains of bacteria thrive in hospitals, endangering any child with an open wound.

Studies have documented numerous cases of horrifying infections caused by circumcision, including tetanus,[10] diphtheria,[11] staphylococcus,[12] streptococcus,[13] bacteremia,[14] septicemia (blood poisoning),[15] meningitis,[16] tuberculosis,[17] and impetigo.[18] In some instances, aggressive and antibiotic-resistant strains of streptococcus have swept through hospital nurseries, infecting every circumcised baby and putting them at risk of serious debility and death.[19] Some infections are so serious that they can spread rapidly to other parts of the body, resulting in umbilical arteritis, phlebitis, and scrotal abscess.[20] Many of these infections have resulted in death.[21]

Even outside hospitals, a circumcised baby is at risk of grave infection. Because babies wear diapers, the raw wound is exposed to fecal material and urine.

I will never forget the time when a baby was brought to my office for his first visit. Two days earlier, the poor baby had been circumcised in a nonhospital setting. The baby was suffering from pseudomonas auroginosa sepsis, originating from the circumcision wound. This is a grave medical emergency, frequently leading to death. The parents had no idea that anything was wrong. The circumciser had convinced them that everything was normal. I immediately admitted the baby to the hospital, where he stayed in the intensive care unit for ten days. The baby almost died. What a terrible way to begin life!

A Circumcision Infection Nightmare

To give you an idea of how serious infections of the circumcision wound are, let me tell you the story of Jacob Sweet.

Jacob Sweet was born on January 16, 1986, at Sisters of Providence Hospital in Anchorage, Alaska. His pediatrician examined him the day of his birth and found him to be a normal, healthy infant. The following day, another doctor took Jacob away and circumcised him without providing Jacob's parents with any information on the normal penis, the risks of circumcision, or allowing them to give informed consent to the surgery.

After Jacob and his mother, Beverly, were discharged from the hospital, the baby developed an infection at the site of the circumcision wound. He began to suffer from vomiting. His parents immediately took him to the emergency room, where it was determined that he had a localized infection in his penis. He was hospitalized in the pediatrics ward for intravenous antibiotic therapy, but was soon transferred to the intensive care ward.

Jacob went into convulsions. In his mother's arms, he involuntarily arched his back, rolled his eyes to the back of his skull, and turned red. He suffered these convulsions every forty-five minutes. Meningitis-causing bacteria had infected his circumcision wound and invaded his brain.

The doctor put the child on an apnea monitor. The monitor sounded several times during the evening. Rather than respond to the alarm, the on-duty nurse turned down its volume to avoid disturbing other patients.

At one A.M., Jacob began suffering brain seizures. Jacob sustained severe and permanent brain damage as a result of his prolonged seizures. Circumcision turned this normal and healthy infant into a severely retarded, blind, and spastic quadriplegic.

At the first trial, Jacob's parents sued the hospital and the physicians for malpractice and lack of informed consent. They explained that they would never have consented to the circumcision if they had been told that the surgery was unnecessary, caused pain, and had risks. To make matters worse, the hospital either hid or destroyed all the evidence associated with the case and then claimed to have "lost" all of Jacob's medical records.[22] Unbelievably, the jury returned a verdict in favor of the doctors and the hospital. Jacob's parents were ordered to pay $150,000 in attorneys' fees to the hospital, the physicians, and the circumciser. Jacob's parents appealed, and, in 1995, the State Supreme Court remanded the earlier verdict.[23]

Jacob requires twenty-four-hour care. For years Jacob's parents have had to pay for this out of their own pocket. Legal and medical malpractice attorney Mark Johnson, who ultimately represented the Sweets in a successful lawsuit against the attorney who bungled the first case, said, "To me the Sweets are heroic figures. . . . They confronted two of society's most powerful institutions: the medical system and the legal system. They fought for thirteen years until they prevailed."[24]

Jacob's father, Gary, has written the following note:

It's so hard for me to put my thoughts down. Our son will grow to be a man in a wheelchair, he is blind, he may never speak, he may never say "Mommy, Daddy," or "I love you."[25]

Gangrene

As a complication of infection, gangrene is one of the most distressing and tragic consequences of circumcision. It is a risk that every baby is forced to run if he is subjected to circumcision. The medical literature overflows with case reports of American babies who were circumcised in first-rate hospitals but who nonetheless contracted gangrene.[26] Gangrene is also a high risk of ritual circumcisions that take place outside of hospitals.[27]

Often called necrotizing fasciitis or Fournier's syndrome, the malevolent bacterial organisms that cause gangrene can easily enter the large raw circumcision wound. Features of this infection include edema (swelling), necrosis (tissue turns black and dies), partial liquefaction of subcutaneous fat, superficial fascia, and the superficial layer of the deep fascia; sepsis; disseminated intravascular coagulation; and hypotension. Mortality ranges from 13 to 60 percent, with better survival seen with more radical surgical treatment.[28]

The treatment for circumcision-caused gangrene is horrific. All of the affected tissue must be cut away. This can leave the baby with an enormous chunk of his groin and abdomen without any covering of any kind. The penis and scrotum are usually destroyed. Emergency skin grafts have been necessary to save babies' lives. Can you think of a good enough reason to subject a baby to a risk like this?

Necrosis

Necrosis means that the penis *dies* and drops off as a result of circumcision. This terrifying nightmare has frequently been reported in the medical literature. One cause of necrosis is *ischemia*, that is, lack of blood.[29] Since circumcision severs some of the important arteries that nourish the glans, infections can easily arise, resulting in death of the glans. Blood flow may also be interrupted by anesthetic solutions containing epinephrine, from vigorous attempts to stop bleeding with suture or electrocautery,[30] or from the prolonged use of a tourniquet, or from a tight bandage.[31] Necrosis is particularly likely to occur if the electrocautery beam comes into contact with a metal circumcision clamp like the Gomco clamp.

In a famous 1966 article, Dr. John M. Foley related the following disasters:

> *As a result of circumcision, some infants die. Countless thousands are doomed to become sexual cripples. In 1958, a 4-year-old boy underwent surgery for an undescended testicle. The surgeon, noticing that the child still had his foreskin, just couldn't pass up this tidbit. The circumcision failed to heal, and 5 days later the penis sloughed off. The parents sued for $150,000 and settled for $80,000. In a similar case last year, the parents asked for $4,500,000. These are two cases that have come to public attention only because of lawsuits.*[32]

Necrosis is far more common than we would like to think. Is this a risk you would want to inflict on your precious child?

Balanitis Xerotica Obliterans (BXO) Secondary to Circumcision

Balanitis xerotica obliterans, also known as *lichen sclerosus et atrophicus,* is a mysterious and very rare disease that forms hard, white, scarlike plaques on the skin.[33] It is thought to heighten a man's risk of penile cancer. Although circumcision advocates claim that circumcision prevents this rare disease, the medical literature presents cases in which BXO has been the result of circumcision![34] I will explain BXO in more depth in Chapters 8 and 10.

Urinary Tract Infection (UTI)

Circumcisers have been relatively successful at making people believe that circumcision prevents urinary tract infections. The so-called studies that they use to try to prove this claim have serious methodological flaws. The statistics are manipulated. Children who should be excluded from such studies have been improperly included, and pertinent information is omitted. Even still, the best they can claim is a tiny fraction of a difference in UTI rates between intact boys and circumcised boys. In Chapter 8 we'll take a detailed look at this topic.

Other studies in the literature, however, demonstrate that circumcision itself is associated with an elevated risk of UTI.[35] This makes sense because the amputation of the foreskin leaves the glans and meatus open and vulnerable to infection. Without the foreskin, the door is left wide open for bacteria to invade and colonize the urinary tract.

Urinary Retention

Urinary retention is the inability of the baby to urinate when he needs to. It is a frequent complication of circumcision that often goes unnoticed.[36] Circumcision-caused urinary retention is a dangerous condition and has been the direct cause of abdominal distension[37] and kidney failure.[38] Often, the cause is the tight circular bandage used to stop the bleeding after circumcision.[39] It is obvious that a genitally intact child is free of any risk of urinary retention because his penis is free of any bandages.

Meatal Ulceration

Because circumcision leaves the glans and its delicate urinary opening (the meatus) unnaturally exposed and vulnerable, a number of problems can arise. One is the ulceration of the meatus,[40] caused by the delicate mucosa of the meatus being burned by urine in the diapers that has turned to ammonia as a result of bacterial action. Basically, meatal ulceration is a severe case of diaper rash.

Meatal ulceration may develop during the first year of life because the glans is no longer protected by the foreskin. This progressive injury is rarely, if ever, seen in an intact boy.

Meatal Stenosis

Meatal stenosis is a pathological consequence of circumcision,[41] characterized by the scarring and contraction of the urinary opening of the glans (the meatus). Meatal stenosis makes urination difficult, painful, and, if left untreated, almost impossible. One of the largest studies ever conducted on meatal stenosis found that 60 percent of circumcised adults suffer from some degree of meatal stenosis.[42]

There are two possible explanations for its occurrence. Amputation of the protective foreskin exposes the delicate mucosa of the meatus to the constant forces of trauma and friction from underwear and harsh chemicals from diapers or laundry detergent. The meatus becomes inflamed, infected, and ulcerated. Eventually, scar tissue develops as the ulcers heal.

Another reason for meatal stenosis is that the destruction of the frenulum and the loss of the blood supply from the frenular artery cause the meatus to be starved for nourishment.[43] The delicate meatal tissues die and are replaced by scar tissue. This causes the urinary opening to become progressively smaller.

Meatal stenosis can be treated by meatal dilation, or more commonly by meatotomy, a surgical operation in which the scar tissue around the urinary opening of the glans is sliced open with a scalpel.[44] Following the operation, a plastic dilator is inserted into the urinary opening several times a day to prevent the edges of the incision from adhering to one another, a procedure that causes additional pain and trauma to the child.

It is important to realize that meatal stenosis would be *entirely preventable* if parents would protect their children from circumcision. One of the functions of the foreskin is to protect the urinary meatus.

Urethral Fistula

A fistula is an abnormal tubelike passage in a body part, resulting from a disease, deformity, or injury. Urethral fistulas have been reported following circumcision.[45] Most have occurred because of either a circumcision clamp or as a result of the Plastibell. In other cases, fistulas have been created by stitches that were used to control arterial hemorrhage in the area of the arterial frenulum.

These fistulas are created because the urethra is actually pulled into and crushed by the circumcision clamp. They may also be the result of a knife or suture. It is difficult for circumcisers to prevent this accident from happening. Circumcisers have difficulty seeing what they are doing when using a clamp. They may also be unaware that a fistula is slowly being created by the Plastibell circumcision device after the baby has been taken home.

Hypospadias and Epispadias

These are usually congenital conditions. Hypospadias is a birth defect in which the urinary opening appears along the underside of the penis rather than at the tip of the glans (the head). Epispadias is a similar birth defect in which the urinary opening appears along the top of the shaft of the penis instead of at the tip of the glans. Both hypospadias and epispadias have inadvertently been caused prior to the application of the clamp or Plastibell.[46] The circumciser inflicts this serious injury by splicing open the glans penis at the time of the dorsal or ventral incision. Similarly, circumcisers have inflicted deep lacerations into the shaft skin or scrotum during this stage of the operation.[47]

Lymphedema

Lymphedema is a swelling of the skin caused by a blockage of the lymphatic vessels or lymph nodes and the accumulation of large amounts of lymph fluid in the damaged region. Lymph is the clear fluid that is collected from the tissues throughout the body, flows in through lymphatic vessels, and eventually drains into the veins. If you have ever had a wound, you may have noticed the clear fluid that sometimes flows from it after the blood has ceased flowing. Lymphedema of the penis may occur following circumcision because the lymph vessels that flow through the skin of the penis and foreskin have been severed and are now blocked by scar tissue. Lymph fluid flows into the tissues of the penis but cannot flow out. The swelling may be especially bad if the circumcision wound separates or becomes infected.[48] The treatment of this complication may require skin grafting.

Complications from Anesthesia

Many parents believe their child can be anesthetized during circumcision, but this is very risky. General anesthesia, in which the child is put to sleep, is very dangerous for a baby and has led to circumcision-related deaths.[49]

One type of local anesthesia sometimes used in circumcision is dorsal penile nerve block. This means that an anesthetic such as lidocaine or prilocaine is injected with a needle into the top (the dorsal side) of the penis. The intention is to inject the anesthetic directly into one of the large dorsal nerves that run down the length of the skin of the penis and partially provide the foreskin with sensation. Unfortunately, it is difficult for doctors to know whether they have injected the anesthetic into the nerve. Also, this type of anesthesia during circumcision has caused many serious complications.[50] When local anesthetic agents are injected too deeply and pool in the spongelike erectile bodies of the penis (the corpora cavernosa), they can damage the tissues, resulting in erectile dysfunction. Additionally, overdoses of analgesia or anesthesia can even result in death.

Another type of local anesthesia that circumcisers are sometimes encouraged to use during circumcision is the direct application of anesthetic creams to the penis. The surgeon spreads the cream inside and outside the foreskin and hopes that the anesthetic will be absorbed by the skin before he starts cutting. The most common anesthetic cream is called EMLA. The manufacturer of this cream admits that it is unsuitable for surgery. EMLA is more appropriately used for mildly painful procedures, such as hypodermic needle injections or the professional removal of unwanted hair through electrolysis.

In August 1994, a Canadian hospital issued a strong warning against the use of prilocaine and EMLA cream upon newborns. A baby in their hospital, a few hours after being circumcised, developed methemoglobinemia, a very serious form of blood poisoning that can cause brain damage and death in small infants. Other cases of methemoglobinemia due to prilocaine have been reported in the medical literature.[51] Lidocaine has caused the same results. Injection of local anesthesia into the penis also has risks, including permanent vascular and nerve damage. The injections can be very painful, and, even when anesthesia is used, the pain of circumcision is still excruciating.

A tragic example of a circumcision disaster happened to two friends of mine, Sam and Judy, who are very good parents. They wanted to protect their newborn son from any pain and trauma, but they were unable to resist the fierce pressure from their parents to subject their baby to circumcision. Arguments revolved around highly debatable but emotionally divisive issues of "heritage" and "tradition." Sam and Judy sought out and found a board-certified urologist who agreed to circumcise their baby. The circumciser agreed to anesthetize the foreskin with "infiltrative anesthesia"—a procedure of injecting a local anesthetic directly into the foreskin before it is amputated. Tragically, the anesthetic distorted the anatomy of the penis in a way that resulted in a surgical mutilation. The baby's glans was permanently twisted at a right angle to the shaft of his penis. The baby required reconstructive surgery under a general anesthetic, which, as all doctors know, is dangerous for babies. The surgery was only partially successful, and the child's penis is still grossly disfigured. I suspect that the boy will need additional surgery when he is older. It is very sad that this poor child may now endure a lifetime of sexual dysfunction, deformity, humiliation, pain, and suffering because of the emotional fears and insecurities of his grandparents.

Vomiting

It was my sad task to publish a case report about a baby who experienced severe vomiting after being circumcised. Following the vomiting spell, the baby stopped breathing and had to be hospitalized for five days so that he could receive intravenous antibiotics. Needless to say, this never would have occurred had the baby been protected from circumcision.[52]

Infants respond to the pain of circumcision by screaming, just as we would if someone slowly crushed and cut off part of our sex organs without anesthetic. When the crying is especially intense, the baby may swallow air. Then, when the mother tries to soothe her baby by feeding him, it may lead to vomiting, followed by apnea.

Apnea (Stopped Breathing)

Apnea is the temporary cessation of breathing. The pain of circumcision is so severe that some babies stop breathing during the surgery. In an important study on the pain of circumcision published in *The Journal of the American Medical Association*, researchers discovered that serious complications occurred during circumcision.[53] One infant experienced the same level of extreme distress as all the others in the study, but two and a half minutes after the conclusion of the surgery, the baby developed an abnormal posture, stopped breathing, and suffered projectile vomiting even though he had been denied food for more than three hours before the surgery. Another baby experienced a choking spell and stopped breathing three and a half minutes after the surgery.

The researchers noticed these serious complications because they were looking for them. One wonders how many babies suffer without anyone taking notice or caring, or even thinking there is anything wrong with projectile vomiting, choking, or cessation of breathing.

Rupture of Internal Organs

Circumcision is so traumatic, painful, and frightening that it literally terrorizes the baby. Some babies have suffered extreme reactions to this experience that few adults could ever imagine possible.

Rupture of the Lung

The medical literature details cases of circumcised babies whose lungs have burst as a result of intense crying. In one case, at Georgetown University School of Medicine, a fifteen-day-old baby with severe respiratory distress was circumcised. He turned blue, started breathing frantically, and cried incessantly. Finally, doctors discovered that the crying had caused the baby's right lung to burst. A drainage tube was inserted and the baby was hospitalized for nineteen days.[54]

Blood Clots in the Lung

A case of life-threatening blood clots in the lung was reported following adult circumcision.[55]

Heart Damage

The serious injury that circumcision can cause to other parts of the body is made clear in reports of babies whose hearts were damaged as a result of circumcision. In one case from Rochester, New York,[56] a newborn baby was circumcised in the delivery room, even though the American Academy of Pediatrics has condemned this practice.[57] The baby immediately turned blue, experienced grunting respirations, his temperature dropped to a dangerous level, and his heart muscle was damaged. This baby miraculously survived, but spent eleven days in the intensive care unit of the hospital.

In another published report, four babies who were hospitalized following circumcision turned blue, were lifeless, had elevated heartbeats, frantic breathing, grunting, and extremely poor breathing.[58] The liver was enlarged in three of the babies, and all babies showed signs of acute heart failure, enlarged heart, and fluid in the lungs. All four babies had been circumcised by the same circumciser, who had tried to control the bleeding with epinephrine solution. The doctors who fought to save the lives of these babies believe that the drug may have induced the chain of events that nearly killed these innocent babies.

Rupture of the Stomach

In Richmond, Virginia, a healthy two-day-old baby was prepared for circumcision by denying him food for five hours.[59] Terrified, the baby began crying hysterically as soon as the circumciser strapped him to the restraining board. After half an hour in this position, the baby vomited. Doctors pumped his stomach. The circumciser proceeded to amputate the baby's foreskin without anesthesia using a Gomco clamp. The baby cried vehemently throughout the ninety-minute ordeal. After the surgery, the baby refused to feed. His abdomen became distended and doctors discovered that his stomach had ruptured, requiring emergency abdominal surgery and the insertion of a feeding tube. After twenty-five days in the hospital, the baby was released. This baby had a perfectly normal stomach when he was born, but the trauma, excruciating pain of circumcision, and his prolonged crying caused his stomach to burst and spill its contents into the abdominal cavity.

Rupture of the Bladder

A five-year-old healthy boy was circumcised by a family doctor who used the Plastibell circumcision device. After the surgery, the boy suffered severe abdominal pains, followed by anorexia, nausea, and vomiting. After forty-eight hours of being unable to urinate, he was admitted to the hospital, where doctors discovered that his bladder had ruptured. The Plastibell device was still in place and had crusted over with blood.[60]

Leg Cyanosis

Cyanosis means that a body part turns blue because blood circulation has been cut off. In one distressing case, a nine-day-old baby was rushed to the emergency room after being circumcised.[61] The baby was in agony, continually cried, and refused to eat. More seriously, his left leg had turned blue, his abdomen was swollen, and his bladder was enlarged. The bandage that the circumciser used to stop the bleeding had been wrapped too tightly, preventing the baby from urinating, thus causing the chain of events. The hugely enlarged bladder compressed the leg veins, thereby interfering with blood flow.

In another published report, three babies suffered cyanosis of both legs following circumcision.[62] In addition to vomiting, restlessness, and refusal to eat, the bladders of these babies became horribly enlarged. Once again, the circumciser caused this nightmare by bandaging the wound too tightly.

Buried Penis

A particularly disfiguring condition referred to as a trapped penis, concealed penis, buried penis, or iatrogenic (doctor-caused) microphallus can occur as a result of circumcision.[63] Circumcision-caused buried penis must be distinguished from the rare and preventable condition of physiologic buried penis, which is a consequence of obesity.

Iatrogenic buried penis can occur for various reasons. First, circumcision is a terrible shock to the body. The body perceives the damage to the penis caused by circumcision as a threat to its survival. The body draws the remaining part of the penis into the abdomen to protect it from further harm. This creates a shorter penis even to the extent that no penis protrudes at all. If the circumciser removes most or all of the penile skin, the raw wound will contract and adhere to the edges of the abdominal tunnel and seal the shaft in a mass of scar tissue.

Correction of the buried penis sometimes involves major surgery. One technique involves cutting two large U-shaped incisions, one on top of the other, across the abdomen. The buried penis is cut away from the surrounding tissue. The edges of the incision are sewn back together transversely to create extra skin to sew over the skinless penile shaft. Another technique involves making Z incisions in the scrotum to provide skin to cover the skinless shaft. Yet another procedure uses inner thigh tissue to provide transplant skin for the penis. These techniques result in massive scarring and loss of function.

Adhesions

Because the glans and foreskin are attached to each other in infancy, the body often heals the circumcision by having the remaining shaft skin—especially if any of the mucous membrane of the inner foreskin is left—reattach to the glans. One study reported that 15 percent of circumcised boys experience these adhesions.[64] Three percent required surgical correction. Many doctors routinely advise parents to tear these adhesions from the glans, causing enormous pain and discomfort to the baby. I advise parents and doctors just to leave the adhesions alone. In most cases, the foreskin stump will naturally detach itself from the glans, just as the whole foreskin would do over time.

Excessive Skin Loss/Denudation of the Penile Shaft

The most common complication of circumcision is the removal of too much skin.[65] Sometimes, overaggressive circumcisers will cut off *all* the skin of the penis, literally skinning the penis alive. This may become apparent only years later. Many circumcised adults complain that too much skin was removed, which can result in painful erections, bowing or curvature of the penis, and hair-bearing skin pulled over the shaft.

I am always saddened when I see a young boy during a routine physical examination for school and notice a flaccid circumcised penis with only a tiny ring of penile skin remaining. The remnant skin is tight and taut, without any loose skin for mobility and coverage, making it physically impossible for these boys to experience a normal and comfortable erection. It is disturbing that this tragedy is so common that many circumcised males grow up never understanding that erections are supposed to be pleasant rather than painful.

Chordee

Chordee is the pathological curvature of the penis. Circumcisers can cause chordee, especially if the circumcision is performed at the time of acute inflammation.[66] It can also be caused, as mentioned above, by the amputation of most of the shaft skin, which tethers the penis during erection, damages the erectile bodies, and causes the production of inelastic scar tissue on one side of the penis.

Cysts

The formation of hard cysts at the circumcision scar has been reported.[67] Dr. George W. Kaplan speculates that these cysts may be produced by the rolling in of skin at the time of circumcision. Some of these cysts can grow to very large proportions. Even small cysts, however, can become infected and may cause local disease. The treatment requires surgical excision.

Skin Tags and Bridges

Another commonly seen adverse outcome of circumcision is the formation of skin bridges between the remnant shaft skin and the glans.[68] In addition to being unsightly and a harbor for the accumulation of debris, the bridges may tether the erect penis, resulting in pain or penile curvature.

There are several factors that can cause a skin bridge. When the glans is torn from the foreskin during the circumcision procedure, the raw surfaces of the glans and foreskin remnant heal together in an inappropriate and undesirable way.

Although unsightly, surgical correction of the skin bridge is unnecessary unless the skin bridge causes discomfort or causes debris to become trapped underneath it. Under anesthesia, the surgeon can cut the bridge away from the glans. Care must be taken because the bridge contains many blood vessels that can bleed vigorously. The raw wounds are treated and dressed to prevent reattachment of the foreskin remnant to the glans.[69]

Pitting of the Glans

Because the foreskin and glans are fused as one structure at birth, circumcision requires that the foreskin be *torn* from the glans. This can cause chunks of the glans to be ripped off with the foreskin as the circumciser forces the metal probe between the foreskin and the glans. Many circumcised males with this pitting disfigurement of the glans have no idea that anything is wrong with them. Since the opportunities for most men to see other penises up close are rare in our culture, circumcised males—regardless of the complications they have suffered—often just assume that they are normal and that other males also have a glans that is pitted and scarred. Pitting not only disfigures the glans, it reduces sensitivity by ripping out the nerve endings that are just below the surface of the delicate mucous membrane.

Plastibell Complications

In addition to an increased risk of infection and gangrene, the Plastibell device is associated with a number of unique, mutilatory complications. If the ring is too small, it may shift and produce an ugly and permanent groove in the glans. If the ring is too large, it may slip down and gouge out a groove in the shaft.[70]

Excessive Scarring and Keloid Formation

A keloid is a mass of raised scar tissue, and a well-recognized complication of surgical and traumatic skin wounds. Keloids are also a complication of circumcision.[71] Most of these cases have occurred to nonwhites, who are more prone to keloid formation. Keloid scar formation is difficult to treat because cutting off the keloid is usually only a temporary solution. Recurrence and exacerbation are likely to occur.

Impotence

Erectile dysfunction has been reported as a result of circumcision in adults.[72] In two documented cases, this complication was caused by injection of anesthetic into the internal erectile bodies of the penis.

Amputation of the Glans

One of the more frequent circumcision accidents is the total or partial amputation of the glans along with the foreskin. The literature is filled with case reports of boys who have been mutilated like this.[73] Part of the problem is that the penis of a baby is small, so circumcisers cannot always see what they are doing. Consequently, they can inadvertently pull the glans into the clamping device, crushing it and slicing it off along with the foreskin.

Reconstructive surgery is required in many cases, but the child will be left with massive scarring. Additionally, no long-term follow-up reports have been published, so we cannot say whether these boys have regained function or use of the glans.

Along with severed nerves and blood vessels, the massive shield of internal scar tissue may permanently prevent normal erection of the glans.

Amputation of the Entire Penis (Penectomy)

Other than penile amputations that occur as part of cancer treatment or elective transsexual surgery, circumcision is probably the single largest cause of penile amputation in the United States.[74]

Accidental penectomy frequently occurs in the Middle East at the hands of barbers during ritual circumcision.[75] Penectomy also occurs just as frequently in American hospitals at the hands of trained surgeons.[76] This tragedy is often caused by operator incompetence, electrocautery burn of the penis, a slip of the knife, or by subsequent gangrene. The true incidence of circumcision-induced penectomy in the United States is underreported due to the medicolegal implications, but if the number of cases reported in American medical journals is any indication, the true rate may amount to at least a half dozen victims a year. The frightening trend in American hospitals today is to subject accidentally penectomized infant boys to "sexual reassignment surgery" and raise them as girls, hoping that they never find out that they began life as perfectly normal boys whose parents were misled by false and biased information and subjected their precious child to this very real danger.[77]

Victims of penectomy, assuming they survive, have lost all penile function and erotic sensation. These boys have been turned into sexual cripples. Of course, even "normal" circumcisions *always* involve amputation resulting in disfigurement, dysfunction, and desensitization. We need to question the motivations of anyone who would try to inflict *any degree* of sexual impairment on our precious children.

Death

There is no question that healthy American babies have died as a result of circumcision. The precise toll of babies who have died at the hands of circumcisers since the program of systematic mass circumcision began is unknown. Likewise, the number of babies that circumcisers annually kill in the United States is unknown, but such deaths do occur. Some brave doctors have risked their professional careers by breaking rank and telling what they know about one of the darkest secrets of the U.S. medical-industrial complex.

These deaths are rarely reported in medical journals. In nations with nationalized systems of medicine, such as the National Health Service in Britain, institutionalized governmental mechanisms for systematic reporting of all related statistics exist. Under such systems, precise figures for the incidence of disease and the incidence of surgical complications can be easily calculated. In the United States, however, no mechanism of equal accuracy or responsibility exists. Rates of surgical complications can, at best, be estimated on the basis of reports in medical journals or random surveys of selected hospitals. Few cases of surgical complications, however, are reported to journals. This is quite understandable. It is difficult to imagine a circumciser willingly reporting to a medical journal how he had killed a baby.

In investigating the deaths of babies killed by circumcision, one must realize that the litigious malpractice milieu existing here makes accurate reporting of such deaths very unlikely. It would take great courage and honesty on the part of a circumciser to report a circumcision death when that circumciser knows that the surgery has been deemed unnecessary by every medical society in the world with a policy about it, and that he may be sued for malpractice.

The most stunning revelation about circumcision deaths came from one of this country's most highly respected and decorated pediatricians, Dr. Sydney S. Gellis, of the Department of Pediatrics at the New England Medical Center Hospital in Boston. Dr. Gellis was honored as a "Pediatric Pioneer" at the 1996 American Academy of Pediatrics annual meeting in Boston.[78] In a famous article in a leading American pediatrics journal, Dr. Gellis revealed that:

> *It is an incontestable fact at this point that there are more deaths each year from complications of circumcision than from cancer of the penis.*[79]

Explaining how circumcision deaths are covered up, Dr. Gellis later expanded his revelation, stating:

> *A number of deaths from circumcision are signed out as deaths due to sepsis [blood poisoning].*[80]

Circumcision deaths are also disguised as deaths due to "complications of anesthesia" without mentioning in the death charts that the baby had been anesthetized for no other reason than for an unnecessary routine circumcision.[81] One way that hospital administrators have tried to cover up these deaths is by omitting any reference to circumcision on the baby's death chart. The deaths are usually blamed on something else. For example, infections that lead to death are generally caused by meningitis,[82] streptococcus infection,[83] systemic blood poisoning, or gangrene. These organisms enter the amputation wound because it provides easy entry rather than because the child is predisposed to infection.

Dr. Robert L. Baker, former rear admiral in the U.S. Navy Medical Corps, estimated that at least 229 babies die as a result of circumcision in the United States every year.[84] Other estimates of the circumcision death rate are smaller, but this is because they are based solely on the number of deaths reported in medical journals rather than hospital records. Nevertheless, it is important to realize that even this "lower" rate is too high for the innocent babies who are senselessly killed in this manner. In a thorough investigation of the medical literature, Dr. David Grimes, of the Family Planning Evaluation Division and the Bureau of Epidemiology at the Centers for Disease Control in Atlanta, Georgia, noted:

> *Newborn circumcision is not innocuous. While the risk of death from neonatal circumcision is small, approximately two deaths per million procedures, the risks of complications range from 0.06 to 55 percent in different studies, reflecting large differences in patient follow-up and in definitions of complications.*[85]

Again, this is hardly the true figure. It is just the figure based on the few reports that have been published in medical journals. Of course, some unethical doctors may say that two or three babies senselessly killed each year is a small number and therefore acceptable. Even one circumcision death, however, is too many when it is *your* baby who has died.

While the number of medical journal reports of circumcision-related deaths is scandalously small, a number of additional cases of circumcision-caused deaths have been reported in the popular press.[86] With heartrending headlines like "Infant Bleeds to Death After Being Circumcised,"[87] "Grand Jury to Probe Death of Baby After Circumcision,"[88] "Boy's Autopsy Results Expected: Five-Year-Old Lapsed into Coma Following Circumcision,"[89] and "Circumcision That Didn't Heal Kills Boy."[90] Americans have been presented with a disturbing piece of reality that circumcisers would hope to deny. None of these deaths were reported to the U.S. Department of Health, Education, and Welfare for inclusion in the *Vital Statistics of the United States.* None of the doctors involved in these deaths reported these cases to medical journals. I think that it is extremely dishonest of circumcisers to deny that these deaths occurred just because no one bothered to publish an account of them in a medical journal.

It would be one thing if circumcision were the best and only weapon against a horrible, highly contagious epidemic disease that was killing innocent people in large numbers. Under these circumstances, a few collateral deaths *might* be justifiable. But circumcision is unable to prevent any disease, and, besides, the diseases that circumcision is alleged to prevent are all related to poor lifestyle choices. Even if you were to accept the statistics waved about by circumcisers, the difference in the rates of disease between intact and circumcised males is infinitesimal. The fact that none of these diseases are highly contagious epidemic diseases that kill innocent people in large numbers proves that the killing of even a single baby during circumcision is completely unjustifiable.

Post-Traumatic Stress Disorder

Post-traumatic stress disorder (PTSD) is a psychological disorder caused by a traumatic experience. According to Dr. Janet Menage, the risk factors for the development of PTSD are present where a person feels powerless to stop what is happening, experiences physical pain, perceives a lack of sympathy in the operator, and has little information about what is being done to his body. Circumcision fulfills all of these risk criteria.[91] Victims of PTSD remain hypervigilant and fearful that the traumatic event could be repeated. They are plagued with terrifying recurring nightmares and flashbacks of the experience that caused the trauma. Typical sufferers are men who experienced horrifying events during war, people who have survived catastrophes, natural disasters, or terrifying accidents. We know that infant circumcision is a terrifying, painful, and traumatic event. Can circumcision cause post-traumatic stress disorder?

In recent years, psychologists have begun asking this question and have conducted studies to find answers. Unsurprisingly, study after study has documented that some babies are so traumatized by circumcision that they have grown up to develop and suffer from post-traumatic stress disorder.[92] Dr. Menage found that the stress levels of some circumcised men were as high or higher than those found in soldiers who had survived the Vietnam War.[93] Interestingly, these men are in otherwise good mental health.

Sadly, there is no way to predict which babies will suffer so much during their circumcision that they later develop post-traumatic stress disorder. The only way to protect your child from this distressing condition is to protect him from circumcision in the first place.

WHO IS MAIMING OUR CHILDREN?

One myth that proponents of mass circumcision frequently voice is that complications, when they occur, are caused by unskilled operators rather than skilled surgeons. In an opinion piece, one circumciser gave his spin on this myth:

> *Circumcision is usually regarded as a simple procedure and is typically delegated to junior members of the medical hierarchy, those with minimal surgical experience. It is performed at odd hours, sometimes late at night, with*

> *minimal supervision. Most complications can be traced to poor technique, infection, and above all, untrained operators.*[94]

There is no published evidence to back up this claim. Indeed, a survey of the tragic complications that have occurred during routine hospital circumcision (rather than ritual circumcision) and that have been reported in medical journals reveals that circumcision-related tragedies are caused by either experienced operators or operators whose skills are undisclosed.

For instance, *The Journal of Urology* recently reported a case in which part of the glans was amputated during newborn circumcision by a "nonurologist specialist with experience of more than 300 circumcisions with the Sheldon clamp and no previous complications." [95]

It may well be true that many circumcisions are performed by poorly trained interns, but it is unnecessary to assume that poorly trained interns are responsible for the majority of botched circumcisions. One ought to question why poorly trained interns would be allowed to perform surgery on the penis in the first place. In any event, the claim that most complications are caused by untrained operators is unsupported by the medical literature. Peer reviewers, however, who should be aware of this easily verifiable fact, have failed to correct this misperception and have allowed such statements to proliferate. By failing to check this myth, circumcisers successfully shift the blame for circumcision complications onto "unskilled operators" rather than on the policy of mass circumcision. In this way, peer reviewers who fail to correct this myth reveal their own biases.

If you are a father, please ask yourself what it would take to make you put *yourself* at risk for any of the complications we have discussed in this chapter. Would any amount of money induce you to part with a piece of your penis knowing that there was a chance that your entire penis could be destroyed, that you could contract gangrene, or bleed to death? If parents were given the facts about these risks and if they were told that the risks far outweigh the supposed benefits, none would choose to put their precious baby at risk of such horrifying complications. My heart goes out to the poor little boys who have been seriously injured in a circumcision accident. I am immensely saddened by all the boys who have died from circumcision and *those who have almost died.* The only logical way to spare your child from these tragedies is to protect him from circumcision.

Chapter Five

• • •

Disadvantages of Circumcision

Circumcision causes pain, trauma, and a permanent loss of protective and erogenous tissue. . . . Removing normal, healthy, functioning tissue for no medical reason has ethical implications: circumcision violates the United Nations' Universal Declaration of Human Rights (Article 5) and the United Nations' Convention on the Rights of the Child (Article 13).[1]

Leo Sorger, M.D.

Surgery can be lifesaving. Indeed, modern surgical advances have reduced the risks and complications of all surgeries. Yet, every surgical operation still has risks and disadvantages. Risks are the accidents that might occur. Disadvantages are the *inevitable* negative outcomes of any surgery. These range from scars and deformities to behavioral problems. Some are minor and hardly noticeable. Others are quite serious. Everyone who undergoes any kind of surgery will suffer from the disadvantages. Circumcision is no exception. Because circumcision became so common in the United States during the Cold War, many people are unable to recognize these disadvantages for what they are. They have been led to believe that these disadvantages are "normal" because most American males underwent the same surgery and they all had part of their penis removed. Nothing could be further from the truth. With part of the penis missing, they are abnormal.

Although the idea that routine infant circumcision has some benefits is extremely controversial, there is no controversy about its many disadvantages. Every baby who is circumcised must spend the rest of his life with these disadvantages. Circumcision is much more than clipping a fingernail, as I have heard one biased physician describe the surgery. If men were permitted the dignity of a choice over circumcision and if they were given the facts about the disadvantages in advance, I sincerely doubt that any man would choose to have part of his sexual organs removed in exchange for the *possibility* that he might experience a benefit of some kind. After weighing the risks and disadvantages against the alleged benefits, ask yourself whether you would sacrifice any part of your own body, risk horrible surgical accidents, and suffer a lifetime of unavoidable disadvantages just on the off chance that you *might* experience a slight resistance to a rare but curable disease that you could have avoided without surgery just by making the right lifestyle choices. I am certain that you will agree that everyone should have the right to make decisions for himself about his own body parts.

There are two kinds of disadvantages: short-term and long-term. The short-term disadvantages are noticed immediately. The long-term disadvantages may appear only later in life. Both, however, are inevitable.

SHORT-TERM DISADVANTAGES

For the baby that has just been circumcised, there are a range of disadvantages that occur with varying severity. In Chapter 3, we talked about the disadvantages that the baby experiences immediately after being circumcised. These may include days—and maybe even weeks—of excruciating postoperative pain. Babies also have their sleep patterns disrupted. They often refuse to nurse at their mother's breast, even with the aid of an experienced lactation consultant.

The shocking thing about these disadvantages is that most parents are never told that they are the negative consequences of circumcision. Hospital staff may wrongly tell the parents that the baby is normal. Parents whose newborn babies were circumcised at birth are often just left to assume that all baby boys behave like this. Objective scientific studies have proven just how wrong this assumption is.

LONG-TERM DISADVANTAGES

Long-term disadvantages are problems that affect every circumcised male. Some are called long-term because they are immediately apparent after the surgery and last a lifetime. Others become apparent only later on in life. All cause noticeable alterations in sexual behavior, sensation, and function.

Hygienic Disadvantages

If the foreskin has been amputated, the baby's penis has lost its normal protective covering. The delicate glans has been prematurely exposed. This organ that nature intended to be an *internal organ* has now been surgically externalized. The little glans is now permanently exposed to feces, urine, and the constant rubbing of diapers. If the diapers are chemically treated, the delicate mucosal tissues suffer prolonged exposure to these irritants. In adulthood, the unprotected glans is constantly exposed to the abrasive effects of clothing and the irritation of chemicals and dirt.

Loss of Penile Skin and Its Sexual Consequences

It is obvious that circumcision amputates skin from the penis. Depending on the size of the boy's penis and the zeal of the circumciser, boys can lose between 50 and 80 percent or more of the skin of the penis. This loss has a number of disturbing consequences.

First of all, normal erections are impossible. In the intact penis, there is always enough skin to fully cover the shaft, plus enough left over to slide up and down the shaft in order to stimulate the penis sexually. After circumcision, this mobility is destroyed. This remnant shaft skin is usually stretched very tightly. Frequently, skin from the scrotum and abdomen are pulled down on the penile shaft. This causes rough, hair-bearing skin to appear on the penis. Many unfortunate circumcised males have no idea that the penis is supposed to be free of hair.

The normal penis hangs gracefully from the body, pointing downward. The smooth, clean line of the uninterrupted shaft skin flows down to the tapered pucker of the preputial orifice. The normal penis also has a wide range of motion.

Another, more serious problem with the lack of skin is that the extreme tightness can cause the penis to bend or curve during erection. This can damage the developing internal erectile bodies, making the curvature permanent.

Without the skin mobility that the foreskin provides, circumcised males have to invent un-biological and anti-physiological ways to stimulate themselves sexually. To try to compensate for the loss of the foreskin, an entire sexual aid industry has sprung up in the United States. Many circumcised males have little choice but to respond to the advertisements in magazines and buy artificial, chemical-laced, factory-made lubricants. After applying the substance to their glans and hand, they use their hand directly on the glans to stimulate it. For many circumcised males, this is a routine chore. They are ignorant of the fact that this is abnormal. It is hardly the way nature intended the penis to be stimulated. They are missing the normal lubricants and natural gliding action of the foreskin.

When the penis is intact, lubricant is unnecessary. The hand slides the foreskin up and down the erect shaft. The foreskin stimulates the glans, and the glans stimulates the rich erotogenic nerve endings in the foreskin. Pleasure also comes from stretch receptors in the foreskin that respond to the repeated opening and closing of the lips of the foreskin as the glans slides in and out. The hand rarely touches the sensitive glans. You see, in the normal, intact penis, the glans is so beautifully sensitive that touching it with the hand is somewhat unpleasant. The penis was never designed to be stimulated this way. It is also rather unhygienic. Unfortunately, circumcised males have no choice but to place their fingers directly on the glans. Another concern is that no studies have ever been published on the long-term safety of using artificial lubricants on the penis.

The loss of skin mobility also affects sexual intercourse. Instead of the muscles in the vaginal wall holding the skin of the penis in place while the erectile bodies slide in and out of their own richly erogenous sheath of skin, the dowel-like circumcised penis must scrape in and out of the vagina like a ramrod. This is hardly the way nature intended the female to be stimulated. The result is dryness, friction, and, if carried on for too long, pain. Many women in the United States suffer from pain during sexual intercourse. I think that it is about time that we recognize that male circumcision plays a significant role in female discomfort and dissatisfaction.

Of course, the sexual aid industry has responded by marketing lubricants to help circumcised males have vaginal sex. Even so, these lubricants are only mimicking (poorly) what the foreskin does naturally and for free. As with the masturbation creams that circumcised males buy, no studies have been performed to determine the long-term health consequences for women from these vaginal lubricants.

Recently, I examined a set of two-year-old twins for their first visit to my office. Their mother told me how the twins had been immediately circumcised after their birth at an army hospital in Texas. She never had a chance to see her babies intact and whole. She never gave her consent to the procedure and was denied her legal right to say that she wanted her boys to be spared circumcision and allowed to remain intact. This fact alone was an actionable offense. To make matters worse, the circumciser removed almost all of the shaft skin from the penises of the boys. The shafts were covered with scar tissue. No loose skin remained to allow the penis to become erect normally and comfortably. I see this tragedy too often in my practice. If more doctors understood how this surgery can negatively impact males for the rest of their lives, I doubt that circumcision would be as prevalent as it has been in the United States.

Damage to the Glans

After amputation of the foreskin, the glans is unnaturally and permanently externalized. In order to protect itself, the artificially exposed mucous membrane of the glans thickens and develops a cornified, horny layer of *keratin* to cover itself. This sclerotic thickening is called *keratinization*. As a result, the glans looses its healthy, smooth, shiny, deep red or purple color and becomes dull, insensitive, tough, and leathery. The nerve endings near the surface of the glans become buried beneath the buildup of thick and dry layers of keratinized tissue. This reduces the sensitivity of the glans and of the whole penis to a large degree. The damaging effect of keratinization on sensitivity of the glans was conclusively demonstrated in a classic study conducted by researchers at the Department of Anatomy at the Pennsylvania State University College of Medicine.[2] The normal glans is covered only by a very thin layer of mucosal tissue. The nerve endings are just below this. Only the soothing and protective presence of the foreskin can prevent the glans from degenerating like this.

Because they have never known life any other way, many males who were circumcised at birth have trouble understanding this damage. All they know is what they have. They have no memory of what their penis was like before it was circumcised. They have nothing to compare it with. Many force themselves to believe that they have all the sensation they could ever want. This is like a color-blind man convincing himself that there is no such thing as color vision and that he can see perfectly with his eyes just as they are.

Circumcisers, however, cannot deny that the glans becomes keratinized after the amputation of the foreskin. Since they cannot deny it, they now claim that it is an advantage. Some even stoop to the absurdity of calling the normal penis "poorly keratinized." This is like calling a woman with an unblemished complexion "poorly pockmarked."

Infliction of a Scar

Every circumcised penis has been scarred. A circumferential scar runs around the shaft of the penis. It marks where the two cut edges of the foreskin stump were crushed and mashed together. The Plastibell method of circumcision leaves a more prominent and darkly colored scar. Other methods leave a jagged, uneven scar.

In the normal penis, the shaft skin and the foreskin are the same hue because the foreskin is an extension of the shaft skin. There is no dividing line between them. This gives the normal penis a smooth, clean, streamlined appearance. In males with more darkly pigmented skin, circumcision creates a more prominent scar. It also gives the remnant skin on the penis a startlingly unnatural two-toned appearance. The remaining mucosal tissue from the foreskin that has been pulled down onto the shaft just behind the glans is stitched or crushed to meld with true shaft skin. Depending on how aggressively the circumciser cut the penis, this scar can be anywhere along the shaft, sometimes even immediately near the place where the penis joins the scrotum. The shaft skin is darker than the damaged mucosal tissue. A circumcised penis in this condition looks even stranger and is more noticeable than in males who have fairer skin.

Decrease in Sexual Sensitivity of the Whole Penis

It should be obvious by now that circumcision dramatically reduces the sensitivity of the penis, but what does this mean exactly? It means that the quality and quantity of erotic sensations that the remnant penis is capable of conveying to its owner are sharply reduced. In addition to all the nerve endings in the foreskin that are destroyed forever, the nerve endings in the glans are damaged and buried under layers of cornified keratin.

Additionally, the range of sensations is acutely reduced. The sensations that the foreskin conveys when its lips open and when the glans stimulates it are very different from the sensations of the glans. You can demonstrate for yourself the difference. Wet your lips and lightly stroke them with a finger. Now, stroke your chin. Notice how different the sensations are. The lips are invested with Meissner's corpuscles, just like the fore-skin. The chin, however, is devoid of Meissner's corpuscles.

Try another experiment. Take a pin. Gently press the tip of the pin into the palm of your hand. Notice how quickly you feel the pin. Now, press the same pin into the back of your hand. Here, you will notice that you have to push the pin harder to feel anything.

Finally, to give you an idea of the range of sensations pro-duced by the lips of the foreskin, gently kiss the back of your hand. Which body part is more stimulated: your hand or your lips? The answer is that your lips are feeling a greater range of sensations. They are better at detecting texture, temperature, and light touch. Slide your lips along the back of your hand. Notice how well they detect the presence of hairs, bumps, and the placement of bones beneath the skin. This is almost as high as the level of sensitivity that the lips of the foreskin are capable of experiencing.

Sadly, these natural and normal means of experiencing the world are entirely lost to the circumcised male. The foreskin produces an entirely different range of sensations than the glans. Circumcision entirely destroys them. The glans is still a won-derful organ, but it is simply unable to duplicate the sensations of the foreskin. Together, the foreskin and glans complement each other. They work with each other to produce a symphony of sensation and feeling. To extend this musical analogy, a Beethoven violin sonata would be less beautiful with just the piano accompaniment. You need the violin to get the full flavor of the composition.

Looking Different from Most Other Males in the World

Circumcision dramatically alters the appearance of the penis. In our world, most males are intact. Circumcision is primarily found among some Third World tribes in Africa, among Muslims, and among Jews. Together with the industrially circumcised males of the United States, approximately 15 percent of the male population of the world has undergone circumcision. In the other countries of the world, such as the nations of Europe, circumcision is unknown except among Muslim immigrants and small Jewish minority communities.

What does this mean for your American child? It means that circumcision brands him. It permanently marks him as being different from his peers in the rest of the civilized world. It cuts him off from the heritage of his ancestors. Circumcision, however, is unable to stamp him as an "American." On the contrary: The great Christian heroes of American political and popular history were all intact. George Washington, Thomas Jefferson, Abraham Lincoln, Teddy Roosevelt, General Douglas MacArthur, Ronald Reagan, Elvis Presley, Clark Gable, Gary Cooper, et al. were all intact. Circumcision insidiously and unfairly brands our American boys as having been processed through the cold, impersonal, unfriendly, circumciser-dominated, globalized, medical-industrial complex.

The medical systems of the most prosperous European countries are just as good as, and, in many cases, superior to the medical system in the United States. Doctors in Europe have looked at all the so-called studies that American circumcisers hold up as proof that they have a right to interfere with and cut away at the private parts of our American boys. European medical experts have rejected these "studies" as ludicrous and have condemned circumcision as barbaric. For them, these pro-circumcision "studies" and ideologies are motivated by the same primitive and dark compulsions that lead some doctors in Egypt and elsewhere in the Third World to produce "studies" allegedly proving that female circumcision is medically necessary and beneficial.

A few years ago, I had dinner with a very famous Swedish pediatrician who was visiting Los Angeles. We spoke of many medical subjects, ranging from breast-feeding and natural childbirth to medications and the treatment of otitis media (ear infection). When the subject of circumcision came up, he paused and looked very puzzled, saying, "Why, oh why, do Americans do such a thing?"

Circumcised Americans are usually shocked to discover that the males in the rest of the civilized world are genitally intact. It is often during a trip abroad that the average American male discovers for the first time that part of his penis had been cut off. One young American college student told me of his emotionally traumatic experience related to having a European roommate in his college dorm. This American had never seen an intact penis before! No one had ever told him that part of his penis had been amputated shortly after his birth. When the roommate explained what the foreskin is and how it operates, this American student was deeply disturbed and troubled. It had never occurred to him that he had spent his entire life unaware that part of his penis was missing. He realized how unfair it was that a circumciser had cut off part of his body without asking his permission. He realized that he would *never* have consented to allowing anyone to cut off any part of his penis for any reason. It was also at this time that this American college student noticed that he had an ugly brown circumcision scar running around the shaft of his penis. He had previously assumed that all boys were born with this sort of marking. He thought the scar was normal, rather than the result of surgery.

It is unfair for any child to be branded like this without his permission. It is unfair to take a child and literally *cut him off* from his human heritage and oblige him to spend the rest of his life suffering or putting up with the disadvantages that I have listed in this chapter. Each and every one of us deserves the opportunity to enjoy our birthright to a God-given, intact, fully functioning body. I believe that America is waking up to these important facts. This is why increasing numbers of Americans are saying "No!" to circumcision and protecting their babies' birthright to an intact body.

Chapter Six

●●●

Circumcision in Religion

There is no reason for tying circumcision to a humanistic Jewish birth celebration. Despite its historic importance, it is simply inappropriate in the same way that female segregation is inappropriate.[1]

Rabbi Sherwin T. Wine

Watch out for those wicked men—dangerous dogs, I call them—who say you must be circumcised to be saved. For it isn't the cutting of our bodies that makes us children of God; it is worshiping Him with our spirits.

St.Paul (Philippians 3:2–3)

Americans take religion very seriously. Our nation was founded by deeply religious groups who came to these shores from Europe to worship in freedom and according to their own conscience. While circumcision was never a part of the religion of this country's founders, a few groups have settled here whose religious traditions include the blood rite of penile circumcision. Let us examine the religious reasons for circumcision and see if we can fit them into an ethical framework.

CHRISTIANITY

If you are a Christian, you are entirely free of any religious reasons for circumcision. In fact, historically, Christians have been specifically forbidden to practice circumcision. I suspect that when some misinformed Christians imagine that they have a religious reason for circumcising their children, they are really just grasping for additional excuses to follow the false medical indoctrination they have received their entire lives. Some circumcised Christian males who use this excuse may simply be looking for another rationalization for what unfairly happened to them when they were born.

Christians who mistakenly think that they have a religious justification for circumcision ought to read the New Testament. Here, it is clear that the early Christian Church, under the guidance of St. Paul, abolished circumcision. Throughout his epistles, St. Paul took every opportunity to condemn circumcision, as the following quotations prove:

> Behold, I, Paul, tell you that if you be circumcised, Christ will be of no advantage to you. (Galatians 5:2)

> And even those who advocate circumcision don't really keep the whole law. They only want you to be circumcised so they can brag about it and claim you as their disciples. (Galatians 6:13)

> For there are many who rebel against right teaching; they engage in useless talk and deceive people. This is especially true of those who insist on circumcision for salvation. They must be silenced. By their wrong teaching, they have already turned whole families away from the

truth. Such teachers only want your money. (Titus 1:10–11)

It is true that Jesus was probably circumcised, but this is because his parents were Jews. Jesus was denied any choice in the matter. Besides, Christians are hardly required to copy everything that happened to Jesus. Jesus never advocated circumcision. After all, the earliest Christians—the ones who actually walked with Jesus—abolished circumcision. And they did it for good reason.

What did Jesus think about circumcision? In the fascinating apocryphal Gospel of Thomas, Jesus is asked by his disciples about circumcision:

> *His disciples said to him: Is circumcision useful or not? He said to them: If it were useful, their father would beget them from their mother (already) circumcised. But the true circumcision in the Spirit has proved useful in every way.*[2]

The founders of Christianity believed that God himself condemned circumcision as a blasphemy invented by foolish men. The New Testament Apocryphal Book of Esra reports the word of God, which came to Esra, the son of Chusis, in the days of Nebuchadnezzar thus:

> *When you bring offerings to me, I will turn my face from you; for your feasts and new moons and circumcisions of the flesh have I not asked.*[3]

Early Christians took the abolition of circumcision very seriously, and the early Church quickly passed laws banning circumcision under penalty of death. The original Church laws against circumcision read:

> *Roman citizens, who suffer that they themselves or their slaves be circumcised in accordance with the Jewish custom, are exiled perpetually to an island and their property confiscated; the doctors suffer capital punishment. If Jews shall circumcise purchased slaves of another nation, they shall be banished or suffer capital punishment.*[4]

The Church was also very concerned about Jews circumcising Christians or citizens of any other sect. Consequently, they passed laws protecting people from such an assault. The Church law states:

> *Jews who circumcise a Christian or commit him to be circumcised, their property shall be confiscated and they shall be perpetually banished.*[5]

All forms of sexual mutilation—both circumcision and castration—have been banned by the Church as insults to God. According to the teachings of the early Church, circumcision is *blasphemy* because it implies that God made a mistake when He created the human body. The Apostolical Canons of the Church state:

> *Canon XXII*
> *He who has mutilated himself, cannot become a clergyman, for he is a self-murderer, and an enemy to the workmanship of God.*

Canon XXIV
If a layman mutilate himself, let him be excommuni-
cated for three years, as practicing against his own life.[6]

The enlightened holy men who worked hard to establish, spread, and safeguard Christianity strongly condemned circumcision. These were the early Fathers of the Church, such as St. Augustine, who wrote:

> *Accordingly, when you ask why a Christian is not circumcised if Christ came not to destroy the law, but to fulfil it, my reply is, that a Christian is not circumcised precisely for this reason, that what was prefigured by circumcision is fulfilled in Christ. Circumcision was the type of the removal of our fleshly nature, which was fulfilled in the resurrection of Christ, and which the sacrament of baptism teaches us to look forward to in our own resurrection. The sacrament of the new life is not wholly discontinued, for our resurrection from the dead is still to come; but this sacrament has been improved by the substitution of baptism for circumcision, because now a pattern of the eternal life which is to come is afforded us in the resurrection of Christ, whereas formerly there was nothing of the kind.*[7]

The other great Church Fathers, such as St. Cyril,[8] St. Jerome,[9] John Chrysostom,[10] St. John of Damascus,[11] St. Justin Martyr,[12] Lactantius,[13] Origen,[14] Tertullian,[15] and St. Ambrose,[16] reaffirmed the ban on circumcision for Christians. Origen said quite plainly:

> *The rite of circumcision . . . which began with Abra-*
> *ham . . . was discontinued by Jesus, who desired that His*
> *Disciples should not practice it.*[17]

Speaking of circumcision, St. Ambrose wisely observed:

> *Nature has created nothing imperfect in man, nor has*
> *she bade it be removed as unnecessary.*[18]

Over the centuries, the Catholic Church has passed many laws
banning the circumcision of children and adults.[19] Martin
Luther preached against circumcision on many occasions.[20]
Even more recent branches of Christianity have taken a firm
stand against circumcision. For instance, the holiest scriptures
of the Mormons, the Book of Mormon[21] and the Doctrine and
Covenants,[22] both condemn and forbid circumcision. Thus, the
traditional Christian response to circumcision has been to reject
it as an insult to the wisdom of God in designing the human
body.

JUDAISM

When most people think of religious circumcision, they think
of the Jews. Circumcision is a deeply sensitive topic for Jews,
but the history of circumcision among the Jews is more varied
and interesting than most people realize.

For centuries, many, and perhaps most, *but not all,* Jews
have been circumcising their newborn boys on the eighth day of
life in a ritual called the *bris milah*—the "covenant of cutting."
Most Jews in the United States, however, have abandoned the
ritual. They just have their children circumcised shortly after
birth in the hospital. Oddly, according to many Jewish religious

authorities, hospital circumcisions are devoid of religious meaning. Consequently, they can be considered as religiously invalid.

What purpose does a ritual circumcision serve? There are a variety of answers to this depending on whom you ask. Many Jews point out that circumcision is unnecessary to be considered a Jew. Jewish law confirms that every child is considered Jewish as long as he is born of a Jewish mother. It makes no difference if he is circumcised or not. Jewish identity is hardly confirmed by circumcision. After all, it is unnecessary for Jewish females to have part of their sex organs removed in order for them to identify as Jews. These fears are common but baseless. I know of many fine Jewish boys who have been warmly accepted into their religious community and have even had a bar mitzvah without ever having been circumcised.

Traditional Jewish circumcision is performed by a ritual circumciser, called a mohel, on the eighth day after the child's birth. The ritual surgery is performed at home, in public, but females are generally excluded from observing the actual cutting. They will usually wait in another room where they are unable to hear the baby's screams of pain and terror. The men may crowd around the baby with extreme interest as the infant loses what they lost. They raise their glass of schnapps to toast the idea that he will now be surgically altered to look like other "members of the tribe." They may attempt to drown out the baby's screams with chanting.

For many Jews, the *bris milah* is a joyous occasion when friends and family come together for a feast and celebration to welcome the new member of the family. The guests will eat, drink, and raise toasts to honor the valuable son. Ironically, everyone celebrates except the new son. I can understand why many Jews place such a high value on the *bris milah* ceremony. It is a beautiful idea to welcome a new baby with holy celebration. Yet, the actual penis cutting is only a tiny part of the celebration. As I will explain in greater detail later, the positive and affirming aspects of the ceremony can be preserved, enhanced, and enjoyed even if the circumcision is omitted. Reaffirming one's faith and community should be a spiritual process that takes place in the heart. The important thing to celebrate is the *life* of the new baby rather than the cutting of his penis.

Most people assume that circumcision has always been a part of Jewish life. In Genesis 17, we read that the Lord appeared to Abraham when he was ninety-nine years old and made a covenant with him, agreeing that he would be the God of the Jews and the Jews would worship no other god but him. To seal the bargain, Jehovah is reported to have said to Abraham:

> *For your part, you must keep my covenant, you and your descendants after you, generation by generation. This is how you shall keep my covenant between myself and you and your descendants after you: circumcise yourselves, every male among you. You shall circumcise the flesh of your foreskin, and it shall be the sign of the covenant between us. Every male among you in every generation shall be circumcised on the eighth day, both those born in your house and any foreigner, not of your blood but bought with your money. Circumcise both those born in your house and those bought with your money. (Genesis 17:9–13)*

Biblical scholars, however, have known for a long time that this passage was never original to the Bible. It was added about 500 B.C., over one thousand years after the time of Abraham. Scholars David Rosenberg and Harold Bloom have published a full translation of the original version of Genesis, which dates from about 950 B.C. Here, Chapter 17 is conspicuously absent. All we read is that:

> *It was that day Yahweh cut a covenant with Abram: "I gave this land to your seed, from the river of Egypt to the great river, Euphrates—of the Kenite, and Kenizzite, the Kadmonite; of the Hittite, the Perizzite, the Rephaim; of the Amorite, the Canaanite, the Girgashite, the Jubisite."*[23]

As you can see, there is no mention of circumcision as a sign of this bargain. Along with biblical scholars, the only conclusion is that circumcision was never originally a part of Judaism. Why, then, was circumcision incorporated into priestly Judaism?

Rabbi and historian Lawrence A. Hoffman explains that by the late fifth century B.C., at the time of the return of the Jews from Babylonian captivity, the priesthood tried to confirm their status as the dominant political force among the Israelites.[24] They did this by instituting a temple-centered sacrificial cult into which newborn males were initiated by circumcision. They created the Abrahamic circumcision myth and inserted it into the most important part of Genesis, pretending that it had been there all along. The priesthood maintained their grip on power until about A.D. 71, when they were overthrown. Unfortunately, circumcision remained entrenched in Hebrew practice.

Following the destruction of the temple in Jerusalem and the overthrow of the tyrannical priesthood, Judaism underwent major changes. It was now under the direction of rabbis, or teachers. The earliest account of the rules, technique, and method of Jewish ritual circumcision were recorded about A.D. 200 in the Mishnah, a compendium of additional rules and regulations, compiled by Rabbi Judah the Patriarch.[25] These rules are upheld and supported in the Talmud, which is a commentary on the Mishnah.[26] These rules have been observed and fiercely defended up until modern times.[27]

According to the Mishnah, ritual circumcision has three crucial stages; *milah* (cutting), *periah* (tearing), and *metzitzah* (sucking).

The first stage of the operation, *milah*, is accompanied by formulaic incantations. A male holds the baby down while the circumciser grasps the baby's penis and pulls the foreskin through a slit in a metal plate. In one blow with his knife, the circumciser severs the parts of the penis that protrude through the plate.

In the second phase, *periah*, the circumciser inserts a specially sharpened fingernail into the raw wound and proceeds to tear and scrape away the inner fold of the foreskin that still adheres to the glans. The circumciser must tear away every shred of foreskin from the glans. Otherwise, the ritual is invalid.

In the third stage, *metzitzah*, the circumciser bends over the child, takes the bleeding penis into his mouth, clamps his lips around the penis, and actually sucks the blood from the wound. The circumciser performs *metzitzah* several times. Many Jews still say that *metzitzah* is also required and cannot be omitted.

After he has sucked the baby's penis, the circumciser places a lint cloth over the wound. If the baby survives and the wound remains free of infection, cicatrization (scarring) of the raw edges of the wound will take a week or so.

Many Jews would like to believe that the ritual sucking of the penis has been abandoned, and, indeed, many Jewish sects have modified or dropped this unsanitary part of the *bris*. Still, it continues. Jewish writer Jack Shamash described the circumcision of his son in 1998 as follows:

> As the rabbi recited the prayers, he grasped a clip from among the tools on the card-table and put it over the

baby's foreskin, pulled it forward and, with a yank of his knife, the foreskin came off in one clean movement. The baby cried, blood flowed on to his penis . . . The rabbi then bent over the baby and sucked the wound. [roman added] *I know this sounds awful, but it is part of the Jewish tradition. It's supposed to help the healing.*[28]

Actually, nothing could be more guaranteed to *prevent* healing. As a doctor, I can think of no better way to infect the baby with all manner of horrible diseases, including HIV and other sexually transmitted diseases. At the end of the nineteenth century, diseased ritual circumcisers routinely, if inadvertently, infected Jewish babies with tuberculosis by sucking the baby's penis and filling the open wound with their diseased saliva.[29] In addition to spreading tuberculosis, circumcisers regularly killed Jewish babies by infecting them with syphilis[30] and diphtheria[31] through the same means of transmission.[32] Jewish doctors spearheaded a movement to outlaw *metzitzah* and require that ritual circumcision be performed hygienically by trained surgeons. Unfortunately, it met strong opposition from conservative forces, and the practice continues in some religiously Orthodox communities.

Reports of severe medical complications from *metzitzah* continue to appear in the medical literature. The March 2000 issue of *The Pediatric Infectious Disease Journal* reported that two American Jewish infants had been infected with neonatal cutaneous herpes simplex—a potentially life-threatening infection—after having been circumcised and having their bleeding penises sucked by an infected circumciser.[33] The authors of the report warn that sucking of the wounded penis can transmit many potentially life-threatening diseases, such as hepatitis B, hepatitis C, and HIV.

The followers of other branches of Judaism alter the surgical techniques to some extent. Sometimes the blood is sucked up through a glass tube placed over the bleeding penis. Some Jewish religious authorities such as Henry C. Romberg insist that the penis must be sucked in order for the circumcision to be religiously valid.[34]

Over the centuries, Hebrew religious authorities have been very clear about their motivation behind the forced circumcision of Jewish babies. They have never pretended that this is a "medical procedure" or even a beneficial procedure. The great rabbi and scholar Moses Maimonides (1135–1204), who is still revered today as one of the greatest of all Jewish thinkers, was very clear when it came to revealing one of the reasons for circumcision. Maimonides tellingly wrote:

> As regards circumcision, I think that one of its objects is to limit sexual intercourse, and to weaken the organ of generation as far as possible, and thus cause man to be moderate. Some people believe that circumcision is to remove a defect in man's formation; but everyone can easily reply: How can products of nature be deficient so as to require external completion, especially as the use of the foreskin to that organ is evident. This commandment has not been enjoined as a complement to a deficient physical creation, but as a means for perfecting man's moral shortcomings. The bodily injury caused to that organ is exactly that which is desired; it does not interrupt any vital function, nor does it destroy the power of generation. Circumcision simply counteracts excessive lust; for there is no doubt that circumcision weakens the power of sexual excitement, and sometimes lessens the natural enjoyment; the organ necessarily becomes weak when it loses blood and is deprived of its covering from the beginning.[35]

During the nineteenth century, the courageous founders of Reform Judaism in Germany and the United States began the task of modernizing Judaism. As part of their reforms, they sought to abolish circumcision.[36] For example, Abraham Geiger (1810–1874), one of the most distinguished rabbis and scholars of the century, disapproved of circumcision, stating:

> *I cannot support circumcision with any conviction, just because it has always been held in high regard. It remains a barbaric, bloody act, which fills the father with anxiety and subjects the mother to morbid stress. The idea of sacrifice, which once consecrated the procedure, has certainly vanished among us, as it should. It is a brutal act that does not deserve continuation. No matter how much religious sentiment may have clung to it in the past, today it is perpetuated only by custom and fear, to which surely we do not want to erect temples.*[37]

Many prominent Jews disapprove of circumcision and have spared their children from it. The great Sigmund Freud (1856–1939) protected his sons from circumcision. Even Theodor Herzl (1860–1904), the founder of Zionism and the spiritual father of the state of Israel, disapproved of circumcision and protected his own precious son from it.[38] Clearly, there has always been a diversity of views on circumcision among Jews.

Some, like rigidly Orthodox Jews, may deny that circumcision is surgery at all. The Orthodox believe that ritual circumcision is performed solely as a religious rite that no human has any right to question. I have heard them deny that even physicians and surgeons have a right to express any critical opinions on the subject. Sadly, some doctors seem to hold the same view.

In many parts of Europe, Jews now protect their babies from circumcision, and yet they still consider themselves active members of the Jewish community. Throughout the Soviet Union, circumcision was forbidden by law at the behest of politically active Jews themselves.[39] Still, even without circumcision, Soviet Jews preserved their sense of identity. Now that the Soviet Union has disappeared and Jews from these regions have migrated in large numbers to Israel and the United States, the majority are still happy to remain genitally intact and to protect their children from circumcision. It is true that some cave in to pressure to have their children circumcised, but many feel perfectly able to maintain their Jewish identity without compromising the bodies of their children.

Many Jews defend ritual circumcision because of the deep meaning they see in the *bris milah,* the ceremony during which the baby is circumcised. In recent years, though, observant Jews in the United States have developed new traditions to replace the circumcision part of the ceremony. Instead of a *bris milah* at eight days, they celebrate a *bris shalom.* Here, the joyous, beautiful, and deeply moving religious and spiritual aspects of the ceremony are retained and enhanced, but no one gets hurt. The baby is named and presented to the community and his penis remains intact. These gentle ceremonies are increasing in popularity. Jews are able to retain the best parts of their traditions, follow their conscience and their hearts in protecting their baby from unnecessary surgery while still affirming the spiritual ties to their community and history.

Many Jews are reembracing the core fundamentals of Judaism and finding that circumcision is incompatible with these ethical doctrines. Dr. Jenny Goodman has written:

> *In Judaism, and in Islam, the human being is considered to be made in the image of God, and God is conceptualized as perfect. So one could argue that interfering with God's perfect creation is a form of blasphemy. In Judaism*

there is a law of 'Shmirat Ha Guf,' the guarding or pro-
tecting of the body. Body-piercing, tattooing and ampu-
tation are all forbidden for this reason. Further, there is
the Talmudic concept of 'Tsa'ar ba'alei chayyim,' com-
passion for all living creatures. If compassion in all its
fullness were applied to 8-day-old babies, circumcision
would become impossible.[40]

The discussion over circumcision will continue within the Jewish community. Sadly, it is hard for some Jews to accept any improvements that could be misconstrued as criticism of Jews or
Judaism. For many forward-thinking Jews, freeing Judaism
from circumcision is not about criticism; it is about spiritual re-
newal and affirmation.

Books and articles on the subject of Jewish circumcision are
appearing in increasing numbers. Among the best and most
thoughtful are those of scholars and thinkers like Dr. Ronald
Goldman. His bold, passionate, and powerful books and medical journal articles have sparked a lively discussion among Jews
all over the world.[41] His books also contain descriptions and
outlines for the *bris shalom* ceremony.[42] Along with Rabbi Ray-
mond Singer, who composed the preface to Dr. Goldman's book
Questioning Circumcision: A Jewish Perspective,[43] I am confident
that questioning circumcision will benefit and strengthen the
Jewish community.

The following is the text of a statement issued by one proud
Jewish physician to members of his community:

A Letter from Dr. Mark David Reiss to His Community

Dear Friends:

For the past two years I have been struggling with my feelings around the subject of *brit milah* (ritual circumcision). This has primarily evolved from my medical experience and subsequent reading. I have now reached a stage where I wish to share my feelings with all of you. I have prepared a statement which I hope you will read. Any comments or response from you would be most welcome.

B'Shalom,
Mark David Reiss, M.D.

CIRCUMCISION: MY POSITION
Mark D. Reiss, M.D.
9 September 2001

I am a 68-year-old retired physician, a Jew who is an active member of a Conservative synagogue, and a grandfather.

When I was in medical school in the 1950s, almost all newborn males were circumcised. Despite the fact that prophylactic surgery was not generally performed, we were taught that circumcision was the correct and healthy thing to do. It was thought to control masturbation, decrease cancer risk, and help curtail sexually transmitted diseases. We learned nothing of foreskin anatomy and function. Infant nervous systems were thought to be undeveloped and their pain was so trivialized that it was almost ignored. As a young physician, I participated in many circumcisions. Over the years I've witnessed *brit milah* in the homes of friends and family.

I was uncomfortable with the practice, but like most physicians, and like most Jews, I said and did nothing to question circumcision.

Two years ago, as I was about to become a grandfather for the first time, my interest in the subject became more focused. I learned that more and more physicians now realize that any potential benefits of circumcision are far outweighed by its risks and drawbacks. The American Academy of Pediatrics has stated that: "Routine circumcision is not necessary." Whether done by a physician in the hospital, or a *mohel* in a ritual *brit milah,* the procedure has significant complication rates of infection, hemorrhage and even death. Mortality may actually be higher than thought since some of these deaths have not been attributed to circumcision, but listed only under their secondary causes, such as hemorrhage or infection. I've learned of the very important role the foreskin has in the protection of the head of the penis in the infant, and in sexual functioning in adulthood. It has also been shown that the newborn feels pain even more acutely than adults do, and that many of the infants who stop crying during circumcision are actually in a state of traumatic shock. To my amazement, I learned that the USA is now the only country in the world routinely circumcising for nonreligious reasons.

With these overwhelming reasons not to circumcise, I began to look at the practice of ritual circumcision in the Jewish community, and I learned that: circumcision is *not* an identity issue. You do not need to be circumcised to be Jewish any more than you need to observe many other Jewish laws. The bottom line is: if your mother is Jewish you are Jewish, period. Among Jews in Europe, South America, and even in

Israel, circumcision is not universal, and growing numbers of American Jews are now leaving their sons intact as they view circumcision as a part of Jewish law that they can no longer accept. Alternative *brit b'li milah* ceremonies (ritual naming ceremony without cutting) are being performed by some rabbis. Increasing numbers of intact boys are going to religious schools, having *bar mitzvahs,* and taking their place as young adults in the Jewish community.

As a Jewish grandfather, I want to assure young couples about to bring a child into the world, that there are other members of the Jewish "older" generation, including other Jewish physicians, and even some rabbis, who feel as I do. If your heart and instincts tell you to leave your son intact, listen!

ISLAM

One would think that the Muslims could claim that they have a traditional religious reason for circumcision. After all, they are the largest circumcising group in the world. Remarkably, however, the holy book of Muslims—the Koran—says nothing about circumcision. In fact, the word "circumcision" never even appears in the Koran. Strangely enough, many Muslims traditionally circumcise their boys—and some even circumcise their girls—under the false impression that circumcision is required by the Koran. Why does this happen?

The Koran, in fact, is decidedly anticircumcision, as can be deduced from the following verses. Speaking of God, the Koran states:

He created everything in exact measure; He precisely designed everything. (25:2)

He designed you, and designed you well. (40:64)

He created the heavens and the earth for a specific purpose, designed you and perfected your design. (64:3)

He created man in the best design. (95:4)

The Koran even blames Satan for tricking man into altering God's creation:

[Satan said:] "I will mislead them, I will entice them, I will command them to mark the ears of livestock, and I will command them to distort the creation of GOD." Anyone who accepts the devil as a lord, instead of GOD, has incurred a profound loss. (4:119)

Finally, the Koran covers all possible loopholes, stating:

We did not leave anything out of this book. (6:38)

The word of your Lord is complete, in truth and justice. Nothing shall abrogate His words. He is the Hearer, the Omniscient. (6:115)

Say, "Did you note how God sends down to you all kinds of provisions, then you render some of them unlawful, and some lawful?" Say, "Did God give you permission to do this? Or, do you fabricate lies and attribute them to God?" (10:59)

Given all of these positive and genuinely admirable verses from the Koran, why does circumcision prevail among Muslims? Dr. S. A. Aldeeb Abu-Sahlieh, an internationally respected scholar of Islamic law, has published fascinating research showing that, even though the Koran says nothing about circumcision, the controversial apocryphal sayings of Muhammad—the Sunnah—which were written down hundreds of years after his death, contain an alleged recommendation of Muhammad that males and females be circumcised.[44] Many Muslim scholars seriously doubt the authenticity of these sayings, especially in light of the fact that the Koran itself states that it is complete and that nothing has been left out. Nevertheless, it is these sayings that some Muslims point to as the religious justifications for what they do to their male (and sometimes female) children.

Classical Greek historians confirm that some Arab tribes dwelling along the Red Sea practiced a variety of penile mutilations centuries before the birth of Muhammad.[45] The migration of Arab tribes and the spread of Islam through warfare, political domination, and the slave trade have caused circumcision to be spread—by force—throughout Africa and parts of Asia. Many Muslims traditionally subject their children to foreskin amputation around puberty as a cruel test of pain endurance, yet it is becoming more common for Muslims to circumcise their children at earlier ages today.

Although the operation differs from country to country, many Muslim circumcisers are generally barbers. In some Muslim countries, boys are usually circumcised between the ages of seven and twenty. There is usually a ceremony to accompany the surgery, but it is always performed without anesthesia and often with unsterilized, makeshift instruments, such as razors or kitchen knives.

In some parts of North Africa, it was reported in the nineteenth century, the barber dipped the freshly mutilated penis into a basin containing egg white, after which he dusted it with powdered henna or rabbit feces.[46] Should the boy display any pain or discomfort the consequences for him and his family could be severe. Muslim fathers have actually killed their boys on the spot after any displays of discomfort.

Oftentimes, boys are circumcised in large groups as a public spectacle. One can only imagine what is going on in the minds of these unfortunate boys, as their sexual organs are exposed, jeered or *leered* at, and then mercilessly and painfully amputated. In Africa, the most alarming rate of severe complications and deaths occur as a result of circumcision rituals.[47] In South Africa, the alarming toll of teenage boys killed or completely castrated in forced tribal circumcision rituals is so high that the ANC government has recently moved to outlaw the circumcision of boys younger than eighteen. Sadly, tribal chiefs have vowed to defy the law and to continue abducting and circumcising boys by force.[48]

In some parts of the Muslim world, circumcision is more extensive than what usually occurs in the United States and involves the removal of *all* the skin from the penis. Practiced in parts of Saudi Arabia,[49] the aggressive form of circumcision, known as pubic circumcision, skin stripping, or penile flaying, cuts away all the skin from the navel to the anus, including the entire external male genitalia. Hot oil is then applied to the massive wound. Pubic circumcision was reported to have been practiced in Yemen and may still prevail there.[50] The death rate is high and the risk of postcircumcision penile cancer is markedly increased,[51] but remarkably few objections have been raised against this practice.

Like so many of us, Muslims have searched for new justifications for an old practice. Religion must have seemed to be a good enough excuse, especially in an environment where almost everyone was illiterate and no one could verify the accuracy of what the circumcisers were claiming. Nowadays, many Muslims have added borrowed medical excuses to their traditional religious excuses. Interestingly, they use the exact same religious and medical excuses to justify female circumcision in those parts of the Muslim world where this unpleasant rite is practiced.

On a happier note, I am pleased to report that there is a growing movement among Muslims to abolish circumcision. Muslim organizations, such as The International Community of Submitters and the devout Muslim founders of Moslem.org and Quran.org, have taken a firm stand against the unauthentic and unreliable Sunnah and against circumcision, proclaiming:

> *To all true scholars of Qur'an the answer is clear. GOD with his infinite grace did not and would not condone such cruel ritual. This act is not found anywhere in the Qur'an. It is only in such man-made innovations such as "Hadith and Sunnah" that one can find such cruel laws and rituals. It is the authors of these blasphemies that are responsible for these centuries-old crimes done in the name of GOD. All throughout history, laws and rituals have been conjured up and put in place in male dominated societies only to subjugate women, children, and the weak.*[52]

Obviously, in this century, one can worship God in any way one chooses without harming a child. We humans have the capacity to show infinite kindness, compassion, and warmth for the innocent and the weak. A covenant with God to raise your child to do good deeds need never mean that a child must be mutilated in any ancient blood ritual. Christians, Jews, Muslims, and others can free themselves from ancient rituals of mutilation and still be graciously accepted into their communities.

We become model citizens who are worthy in the eyes of

God when we lay down the tools of violence and protect our children's sex organs from surgical interference. This truth is beautifully reflected in the rabbinical liturgy of a *bris shalom* ceremony from 1999:

> *We are gathered together today, in the last year of a century which has given us profound and unprecedented insight into our humanity, one hundred years in which we have learned that each of us is fully human from the moment we are born, able to feel and able to remember all the richness of each and every moment's experience.*
>
> *But this century has also given us the Holocaust, a bloodletting of unprecedented proportion. Given both the insight and the brutality of our century, we are inevitably led to conclude that there must be no more bloodshed in God's name. We continue where Abraham left off: We shall do the child no harm.*

Religion is about living a good life, being accepting, reverent, and respectful. Our most precious investment in our future is our children. Let us honor them by giving them a safe, secure, and loving world where they will be protected from all forms and degrees of harm.

● ● ●

Chapter Seven

The History of Circumcision

Future generations will find it inconceivable that millions of Americans mutilated their babies owing to the influence of a man [John Harvey Kellogg] who . . . was obviously a sadistic lunatic.[1]

Sir Arthur C. Clarke

Circumcision is the strangest operation performed today. No doctor routinely circumcises babies to cure a disease, correct a deformity, or repair an injury. Consequently, routine circumcision fails to satisfy any of the mandatory ethical and clinical requirements that any other surgery must meet before doctors are allowed to operate. Why, then, do some doctors in U.S. hospitals circumcise babies? Why did hospitals ever instruct doctors to start circumcising our babies in the first place?

The reason for this strange way of treating babies can be found in the unique history of medicine in the United States. Babies are circumcised because, since the end of World War II, this has become a routine way of processing newborn babies in U.S. hospitals. The reason that circumcision was introduced and institutionalized in U.S. hospitals is long and fascinating.

The true story may surprise you. It may even shock you. Nevertheless, I hope that it will inspire you to start questioning the way we treat babies in this country.

WHERE DID CIRCUMCISION BEGIN?

Anthropologists speculate that cutting off part of the penis began about ten thousand years ago among Arabian or African tribes living near what would later become the Sahara Desert.[2] In response to major climate changes that affected the food supply in North Africa and the Near East, these peoples became increasingly savage, violent, and barbaric. They began to engage in slavery, war, and rape. They subjugated women, low-status men, and children. Instead of worshiping a gentle and compassionate god or goddess figure, they began to worship a bloodthirsty sky god. They institutionalized child sacrifice as a way of appeasing this god. They sexually mutilated their prisoners of war as an act of cruel humiliation. They sexually mutilated their own children of both sexes.

Sigmund Freud believed that these Middle Easterners began substituting child sacrifice, which was an element of their religious rituals, with child sexual mutilations.[3] Instead of killing their own boys, they would just kill part of them—a most essential part of them: They would cut off the penis and testicles of the boys.

As these bloody religious rituals became more common, Freud surmised that they began cutting off less of the penis. Instead of cutting it all off, they cut off just the foreskin. Perhaps they believed that their bloodthirsty god demanded a sexual sacrifice. Perhaps they thought that sacrificing part of the sexual organs of their children would ward off evil spirits and bring them advantages in war. We cannot really know what motivated these tribes. Practically speaking, the rulers of these tribes may have believed that their slaves would be easier to control after they had been sexually neutralized through circumcision or castration.

Thousands of years later, circumcisions appeared in Egypt.[4] Some Old Kingdom (2649–2134 B.C.) artifacts depict a few slaves and priests as having a dorsal slit of the foreskin rather than a circumcision. The sixth dynasty (2323–2150 B.C.) tomb relief, the Mastaba of Ankhmahor at Saqqara, shows something happening to the penis of a "ka-priest." Some misinterpret this as a "circumcision scene," whereas Egyptologists affirm that the scene depicts a pubic shaving and possibly an impending dorsal slit operation. Around 460 B.C., the Greek historian Herodotus recorded with disgust that the Egyptian priests were circumcised. The pharaohs and all other members of the ruling classes, however, were free from circumcision throughout the long span of Egyptian history.

The ancient Greeks were proud of the fact that they were genitally intact, unlike some of their unpopular neighbors in the Near East. Ancient Greek historians recorded tales of various Middle Eastern tribes who dwelt around the Red Sea. Some of these tribes cut off only the foreskin.[5] Others cut off the glans as well.[6] Still other tribes cut off the entire penis.[7] The Greeks were horrified by these tales.

When the Greeks expanded their empire under Alexander the Great, after 336 B.C., they tried to civilize these mutilating tribes. They banned circumcision and castration wherever they found it. They even tried to stop the practice among the Hebrews. The account of how the Greek ruler Antiochus IV Epiphanes, around 175 B.C., tried to protect Jewish babies from circumcisers is recorded in the Bible, in the first book of Maccabees.[8]

When the Romans took over and expanded the Hellenistic

Empire of the Greeks, they were even more determined to abolish circumcision and castration. The great and noble Emperor Hadrian outlawed castration and circumcision throughout the empire. The Romans were so horrified and disgusted by circumcision and castration that they made the punishment for the perpetrators of either mutilation the same—death and confiscation of all property.[9]

Over the centuries, the Catholic Church has passed many similar laws banning circumcision.[10] As you can see, the traditional Western response to circumcision has been righteous indignation. Westerners must have realized that genital mutilation to any degree is ineffective at eliminating sexual desire and, instead, leads to unhappiness and unproductiveness.

THE MEDICALIZATION OF CIRCUMCISION

During the Victorian era, the medical profession was really quite backward. Doctors had a very weak grasp of epidemiology, anatomy, physiology, and other subjects that are fundamental to an accurate understanding of the human body. Back then, most people died of infectious and contagious diseases like malaria, tuberculosis, meningitis, pneumonia, and diphtheria. Doctors knew nothing of germs. They had little understanding of the true relation between diet and health. Doctors were unable to understand how diseases were spread from one person to another. Doctors, in effect, were powerless to prevent or cure these diseases, which now are so easily prevented or treated.

Yet, doctors falsely persuaded themselves that they really could cure these diseases. They even persuaded patients of this. The standard treatments for any disease were bloodletting, purging, and poisoning with mercury and other toxic compounds. These generally useless and harmful "treatments" were thought to be beneficial, even though they often hastened patients to their death. For any sort of injury, doctors generally just resorted to limb amputations. As hard as it is for us to believe, doctors really thought that amputation and bleeding were beneficial and curative. Simple cases of inflammation, infection, or pain would be treated with surgical amputation of the ailing part without any form of anesthesia. Doctors were unable to imagine any other form of treatment.

Being ignorant of the existence and role of germs in the disease process, doctors invented a number of theories about how diseases were caused. One of the most pervasive theories of disease was that masturbation caused almost all diseases. I know this sounds incredible, but it is true. Doctors convinced themselves that masturbation would damage the nervous system, the brain, the heart, the reproductive system, and all the other internal organs. They wrote books and pamphlets to warn people against this natural human behavior.

You see, virtually every healthy person has masturbated, especially during childhood and the teenage years. We now understand that masturbation is normal and healthy. Victorian doctors, however, would admit only that it was common. With this in mind, doctors could correctly say that anyone with a fatal disease had masturbated. Therefore, they mistakenly argued, masturbation must have caused the disease. This sort of false reasoning was rampant in medicine at this time. It seems hard to imagine that intelligent people could have believed such nonsense, but they did. Few other explanations for disease seemed as rational according to the medical ideology of the time.

Borrowing the idea of circumcision from the example of the Jews, doctors decided that circumcision was a perfect cure for masturbation and all of the diseases that masturbation was believed to cause.[11] Doctors perpetuated the fraud that Jews were immune to masturbation and all the diseases it allegedly caused because of circumcision.[12] Doctors also used circumcision as an especially brutal punishment for masturbation. I hesitate to add that Victorian doctors also employed equally cruel surgical punishments for boys who were accused of masturbation. Some of these medical "treatments" include burning the penis with acid, blistering the penis, shredding the skin of the penis with a knife, cutting the nerves to the penis, vasectomy, and castration. As an illustration of this cruel and unusual attitude toward children, a leading American pediatrics textbook made the following gruesome recommendation to medical students:

> *There can be no doubt of [masturbation's] injurious effect, and of the proneness to practice it on the part of children with defective brains. Circumcision should always be practiced. It may be necessary to make the genitals so sore by blistering fluids that pain results from attempts to rub the parts.*[13]

Little girls were subjected to similar horrors, such as clitoral circumcision, clitoridectomy, and amputation of the labia.[14] Referring to the surgical ways of preventing and punishing masturbation, Jonathan Hutchinson (1828–1913), an internationally respected surgeon, spoke for his generation of doctors when he stated:

> *Measures more radical than circumcision would, if public opinion permitted their adoption, be a true kindness to patients of both sexes.*[15]

Since healthy Christian Americans were genitally intact at this time, doctors should have understood the functions of the foreskin. They knew that it was the most sensitive part of the penis and stated as much in their writings. They understood that the penis is sexually stimulated by sliding the foreskin up and down the shaft. Destroying the mobility of the penile shaft skin, they argued, would prevent boys from masturbating. Victorian doctors knew very well that circumcision denudes, desensitizes, and disables the penis. The horrible thing is that they *wanted* to denude, desensitize, disable, and disfigure the penis. Circumcision was punishment just as much as a bogus "cure."

Because doctors had convinced themselves that masturbation was the ultimate cause of most serious and incurable diseases, and because circumcision supposedly prevented masturbation, they began to think that circumcision was the best cure for these diseases, even if the doctor believed that the patient had never masturbated. Soon, doctors were claiming that circumcision could cure an unimaginably long list of diseases. They began insisting that circumcision could cure epilepsy, convulsions, spinal paralysis, elephantiasis, tuberculosis, eczema, bed-wetting, hip-joint disease, fecal incontinence, rectal prolapse, wet dreams, hernia, headaches, hydrocephalus, nervousness, hysteria, poor eyesight, idiocy, mental retardation, and insanity.[16]

"MORAL HYGIENE"

Many Victorian doctors advocated circumcision for hygienic reasons, but it is clear that the word "hygiene" had a different meaning for them. At that time, circumcisers used the word "hygiene" to denote *moral hygiene* rather than just personal hygiene. Masturbation was incorrectly considered to be an immoral act; therefore, they falsely reasoned, circumcision would improve moral hygiene. Doctors also argued that circumcision would promote moral hygiene by desensitizing the penis with the result that men would be less interested in sex.

This concept later became confused with our current understanding of the word "hygiene" because circumcisers insidiously warned parents that bathing the normal penis would lead to masturbation. To prevent a child from handling his penis during bath time, they advocated amputating the foreskin so that "moral hygiene" would be preserved. As one prominent doctor insisted:

> *The prepuce is one of the great factors in causing masturbation in boys. Here is the dilemma we are in: If we do not teach the growing boy to pull the prepuce back and cleanse the glans there is danger of smegma collecting and of adhesions and ulcerations forming, which in their turn will cause irritation likely to lead to masturbation. If we do teach the boy to pull the prepuce back and clean his glans, that handling alone is sufficient gradually and almost without the boy's knowledge to initiate him into the habit of masturbation. . . . Therefore, off with the prepuce!*[17]

RACISM AND CIRCUMCISION

Another important feature of the medical use of circumcision in the nineteenth century was blatant racism. In order to induce the average white Christian American to accept circumcision, doctors consistently categorized the health and morality of the white male somewhere between the Jew and the black. Jews were held up as being morally and physically superior, and solely because Jewish males were circumcised.[18] This is very strange reasoning and it is worrying that such bigotry was actually taken seriously.

Blacks were considered to be on the very bottom of the

moral and physical ladder. Many openly racist circumcision advocates, such as Dr. Peter C. Remondino (1846–1926), author of a notorious diatribe advocating mass, compulsory circumcision,[19] helped spread the myth that white women were being routinely raped by savage bands of black males. Remondino, who bragged about having circumcised "thousands,"[20] and argued that genitally intact males should be denied health insurance,[21] maintained that state laws to legalize the mandatory circumcision of blacks would resolve the so-called Negro Rape Crisis:

> *From our observations and experiences in such cases, we feel fully warranted in suggesting the wholesale circumcision of the negro race as an efficient remedy in preventing the predisposition to discriminate raping so inherent in that race. We have seen this act as a valuable preventive measure in cases where an inordinate and unreasoning as well as morbid carnal desire threatened physical shipwreck; if in such cases the morbid appetite has been removed or at least brought within manageable and natural bounds, we cannot see why it should not— at least in a certain beneficial degree—also affect the moral stamina of a race proverbial for the leathery consistency, inordinate redundancy, generous sebaceousness and general mental suggestiveness and hypnotizing influence of an unnecessary and rape, murder and lynching breeding prepuce. . . . we never hear of a Jewish rapist.[22]*

Remondino and other influential doctors insisted that the foreskin was the cause of the Negro race's alleged criminal degeneracy and depravity. Using the racist image of the savage, sexually uncontrollable Negro—made dangerous and threatening by his foreskin—as a tool to manipulate white people, doctors like Re-mondino shrewdly frightened white families into agreeing to let them circumcise their children. White families were led to believe that this operation would help distinguish them from blacks and make them more like the allegedly superior Jews.

Remondino advocated the mass circumcision of American males for other reasons as well. In a widely read medical journal, he proclaimed to other doctors:

> *Considering the many reflex diseases that do arise from the presence or existence of a prepuce, and the great diversity and far-reaching consequences of these disturbances, I cannot well see how one can rationally cry down circumcision as not being a most useful and salutary preventive measure. Hydrocele, hernia, hip joint disease, epilepsy, asthma, disturbances of speech or of sight, and a whole category of diseases can often be traced to their origins in some preputial irritation or cause.*[23]

During the late 1890s, circumcision was enthusiastically taken up by the misguided and openly racist eugenics movement and used as a surgical tool under the mistaken belief that the alleged "moral" effects of circumcision would be transmitted from one generation to the next. This was especially true when blacks, alleged degenerates, criminals, and young masturbators were targeted for circumcision. We now know that acquired physical and behavioral characteristics cannot be inherited, but doctors who promoted eugenics preferred to believe otherwise. Additionally, amputation of the foreskin was envisioned as the necessary complement to the sterilizing surgeries of castration and vasectomy. As such, it was included in the package of eugenic surgeries, all of which were supposed to be effective in the cure, prevention, and punishment of crimes such as rape, poverty, alcoholism, and masturbation. Throughout the country, countless thousands of inmates of prisons, insane asylums, orphanages, and juvenile correction facilities were systematically circumcised as a cruel means of controlling their sexual behavior. Circumcision was guaranteed to destroy criminal sexual passion, while "asexualizing" surgeries destroyed fertility, thereby preventing the transmission of undesirable traits.

We have seen how the false science of eugenics led to many of the horrors of the twentieth century, such as the Holocaust. Yet, it is astonishing that eugenic surgeries like circumcision, which eugenicists utilized for the totalitarian purposes of social engineering, have remained entrenched in medical practice. By promoting routine circumcision, doctors today are treating all of our children the way they used to treat criminals and lunatics.

THE INDUSTRIALIZATION OF MASS CIRCUMCISION

Despite the hysteria over masturbation, few Victorian doctors thought that mass circumcision of the newborn was a good idea. Most doctors were satisfied with amputating foreskins just from boys and teenagers who had been caught masturbating. In the twentieth century, however, it was a very small cabal of determined zealots who masterminded the scheme to impose involuntary routine newborn circumcision on America.

In 1914, a New York urologist named Abraham L. Wolbarst (1872–1952) published a manifesto for the mass circumcision of all non-Jewish children.[24] Wolbarst was a well-known surgeon on staff at Beth Israel Hospital and the Jewish Memorial Hospital in New York. Wolbarst was among the first and more influential of the twentieth-century circumcision extremists who are responsible for unleashing mass circumcision on America and trampling the freedoms of the American people.

Wolbarst was furious that the medical profession was growing increasingly concerned about ritual Jewish circumcision because of the high number of deaths and deadly infections that arose from the ritual practice of *metzitzah*—sucking the baby's penis immediately after the foreskin is amputated. Now that the germ theory of disease had been discovered, understood, and accepted, caring doctors realized that Jewish circumcisers were regularly, albeit unintentionally, infecting babies with syphilis, tuberculosis, and diphtheria through this extremely unsanitary practice.[25]

In response to mounting pressure for Jews to abolish *metzitzah* because of the diseases it spread, Wolbarst shrewdly put a new spin on the debate and actually began insisting that circumcision *prevented* the very diseases that it was proven to cause. Instead of circumcision being unsanitary, Wolbarst argued that circumcision was sanitary. Instead of circumcision spreading tuberculosis and syphilis, Wolbarst stridently maintained that circumcision *prevented* tuberculosis and syphilis, as well as masturbation. As a matter of fact, Wolbarst was so horrified by masturbation, that even in the 1930s, he argued that adults who masturbated should be forcibly sterilized and forbidden to marry.[26]

With equal fervor, Wolbarst also insisted that circumcision prevented epilepsy, convulsions, and nervous diseases.

Over the decades, a small minority of well-placed doctors joined Wolbarst's crusade and became advocates of mass, compulsory circumcision of American babies. Slowly, they moved across the face of America, infiltrating our hospitals and maternity wards, spreading their agenda of collectivism through mass sexual surgery.

American parents were bombarded with propaganda designed to subvert their native instinct to protect their children from harm. For instance, in 1941, the best-selling *Parents* magazine published a widely read article by the prestigious obstetrician Dr. Alan F. Guttmacher (1898–1974).[27] A dark and little-known secret about Guttmacher is that, during the 1950s, he was the director of the American Eugenics Society, a powerful group that advocated the forced sterilization of targeted races and people who fell into undervalued social categories.

Just as he targeted the poor for compulsory sterilization, Guttmacher targeted American boys for compulsory circumcision at birth. He triumphantly boasted that circumcision would blunt male sexual sensitivity, as if this were a good thing. He tried to scare American parents into allowing their children to be circumcised by falsely claiming that a baby's foreskin needed to be forcibly retracted every day and the glans scrubbed. His key message was that circumcision would prevent a boy from handling his penis and divert his attention from his genitals. Sadly, many American parents fell for this sort of rhetoric. How many millions of American boys had their foreskins forcibly sacrificed because of this one article is unknown.

Another source of persistent antibiological propaganda was the popular medical works of Morris Fishbein (1889–1976), the controversial longtime editor of the *Journal of the American Medical Association.* Fishbein authored the best-selling home medical book *Modern Home Medical Adviser,* which remained in print from 1935 to 1969. Even though his book was extensively revised in subsequent editions, the information on circumcision remained consistently Victorian. With the determination of a zealot, Fishbein took every opportunity to advocate routine circumcision as a prevention for all manner of diseases and taboo behaviors, including nervousness [28] and masturbation.[29] Fishbein insinuated that:

Frequently children will get into the habit of playing with or pulling at the genitals. Such children—both boys and girls—may be in need of a thorough examination by a competent physician. Not unlikely circumcision or other special corrective measure is needed.[30]

During World War II and the Korean War, militant military circumcisers such as Marvin L. Gerber,[31] Eugene A. Hand, Abraham Ravich, Aaron J. Fink—and many others who are still alive and ruthlessly pushing mass circumcision today—subjected Christian American soldiers to unannounced inspections of their penises. These humiliating invasions were called "short arm inspections." Soldiers who were genitally intact were arbitrarily diagnosed with "phimosis" and ordered to undergo circumcision, sometimes under threat of court-martial. Blacks were especially targeted for surgical abuse of this kind. Dr. Gerber even admitted that circumcision was the most commonly performed surgery in the military—even more common than trauma surgery.[32] And this was during a war! These distinguished and otherwise honorable physicians were obviously more influenced by private tradition, superstition, religion, and medical myths than by any kind of rational thinking or genuinely scientific data.

One of the key players in this dangerous game was Abraham Ravich (1889–1984), a urologist at Israel Zion Hospital in Brooklyn. Ravich was one of the twentieth century's most relentless crusaders for compulsory circumcision of all American males. He invented and popularized the myths that circumcision prevents prostate cancer[33] and cervical cancer in females.[34] In addition to parroting Wolbarst's bogus claim that circumcision prevents penile cancer and venereal disease, Ravich promoted his claim that circumcision prevents cancer of the bladder and rectum.[35]

A little-known fact about Ravich is that he was unsatisfied with the plan to institute compulsory circumcision just in the United States. This failed to go far enough for him. In the mid-1960s Ravich flew to Japan, England, and communist Moscow to advocate compulsory circumcision.[36] Thankfully, the medical professions in these countries rejected Ravich's unwelcome overtures.

Ravich was a ceaseless promoter of the now discredited theory that smegma, the healthy and normal preputial secretion, was a carcinogen. It pleased him to imagine that the foreskin caused cancer in whatever body part it came in contact with. He imagined that there was such a thing as the "smegma virus" that migrated out of the foreskin and infected the internal organs of the man and his sexual partners.[37] All of these ideas are ridiculous and were thoroughly debunked in his lifetime,[38] but he refused to admit defeat and persisted in pushing these falsehoods until his dying day.

Ravich was one of the most active circumcisers to lobby insurance companies in the 1950s to provide coverage for routine circumcision. He also lobbied for insurance companies to penalize genitally intact males and either deny them coverage or charge them hefty surcharges. This sort of backstage chicanery and frank promotion of ethnic discrimination is one of the more worrying aspects of the history of circumcision in the United States.

Popular home medical books, such as the best-selling *New Illustrated Medical Encyclopedia for Home Use* by Dr. Robert E. Rothenberg,[39] spoon-fed the American people these myths and dishonestly presented them as facts. Rothenberg assured parents that anesthesia was completely unnecessary. The absolute authority of doctors over people was emphasized by insistence that the doctor would tell parents if circumcision was necessary for their infant. The message buried in this statement was that parents were forbidden to interfere or make a decision for themselves, and that doctors knew best what would be good for other people's children.

Most distressingly, the campaign to exterminate the American foreskin was inadvertently aided by Dr. Benjamin Spock's best-selling book on child care, first published in 1946.[40] Although Dr. Spock (1903–1998) gave newborn circumcision only a weak endorsement, he did make the mistake of repeating the unscientific opinion that a boy should probably be circumcised if other boys in the neighborhood were circumcised.[41] Dr. Spock was a great doctor, but this misguided and thoughtlessly repeated myth only reinforced the anti-American trend toward collectivism and brutal conformity to non-American values. By simply repeating the current misguided thought of his medical colleagues, Dr. Spock's book exacerbated the growing anxiety among the bulk of middle-class Americans that conformity was more important than the values of rugged individualism and strong personal independence—the very values that built this great country of ours. We should remember that the 1950s was an era of great prosperity but it was also the McCarthy era of loyalty oaths, blacklists, show trials, and political suppression. Many decent, loyal Americans were frightened into conforming to whatever officially mandated mode of living would enable them to blend into the background and avoid standing out. This was an era of mass paranoia about the need to conform. Circumcisers took advantage of these fears and peddled circumcision as a means of achieving conformity. Many parents agreed to the circumcision of their children because they were told that this is what all other parents were doing. To his great credit, Dr. Spock later had the courage and nobility to admit his mistake, to remove the misinformation in subsequent editions of his book, and to speak out against circumcision.[42] For millions of American babies, however, it was too late.

Throughout the 1950s, one by one, with very little opposition, hospitals in the larger cities of the United States silently began instituting policies of mass circumcision for all male babies born there. Prior to World War II, most babies were born in the safety and comfort of home. After the war, mothers were increasingly pressured into giving birth in hospitals. Just as American soldiers formed a captive population, unable to refuse a circumciser's order to undergo circumcision, so babies born in hospitals were easy prey for circumcisers. A baby born at home was safe from interference with his genitals. He was gently and protectively cradled in his mother's warm and loving arms. This beautiful, time-honored tradition of welcoming babies into the world was destroyed as birth became industrialized and turned into a "medical emergency." It took only a single high-placed circumcision extremist in a hospital for the life of every boy born there to be negatively altered—through sexual surgery—forever.

In the 1950s, some profit-driven hospitals instituted the practice of automatically circumcising babies in the delivery room immediately after they were born. With the father banished from the operating room, and the mother groggy and confused by drugs, circumcisers could bank on encountering little resistance to their activities. Circumcisers strenuously defended this practice. They insisted that delivery room circumcision was more convenient for the doctor and economically in the best interest of the hospital. Interestingly, an influential paper, published in a leading medical journal in 1953 by two obstetrician circumcisers—Richard L. Miller and Donald C. Snyder—relied heavily on the writings of Abraham Wolbarst to justify immediate circumcision, enthusiastically arguing that it would prevent masturbation and provide "immunity to nearly all physical and mental illness."[43]

Babies were subjected to circumcision before they were even

examined by a pediatrician or even seen by their mother or father. Parents were rarely told that their baby would be circumcised automatically. Even if they were told, hospital staff insisted that the operation was absolutely necessary for "medical reasons." Circumcisers claimed to have incontrovertible data to prove the absolute necessity of circumcision, when, in fact, they were only acting on their personal bias. Parents who found themselves in such hospitals were rarely if ever given a chance to protect their newborn baby from circumcision. Parents who wanted to protect their babies from circumcision had a very difficult time in this sort of hospital. One father told me of his efforts to protect his own newborn son from circumcision back in the 1960s. The father politely told the doctor that he wanted his son to remain intact. The doctor just sneered at him contemptuously. The father repeated his request. The doctor snarled: "Who's the doctor here? *I'll* decide what is best for your son. Circumcision is mandatory at this hospital!"

The circumcisers established a beachhead in the medical schools and hospital administrations in the 1950s and 1960s, and since then, they have metastasized to the point where they have become the arbiters of sexual health and human sexuality. It is no accident that nearly every illustration of male sexual anatomy in medical textbooks, popular medical books, and even American-produced pornography portrays the penis as being circumcised, without comment, as if it were naturally so. The human body had been censored—both literally and figuratively. Several entire generations of American doctors have been deceived into seeing the human body *not* as it really is but as circumcisers want it to be. The rare picture of a normal human penis with its foreskin intact is invariably pathologically labeled as being affected with "phimosis" and thus in immediate need of an emergency circumcision. Thus, like something out of George Orwell's visionary novel *1984*, the normal human penis has been persecuted, subjected to extermination efforts, outlawed, and silently replaced by the artificially created circumcised penis.

By the third quarter of the twentieth century, the situation was spiraling out of control. Under the influence of a handful of well-placed and vocal circumcisers, corporate-run hospitals worked to increase the rate of newborn circumcision to over 90 percent during the late 1970s and early 1980s. Circumcisers were still insisting that circumcision was necessary to stop masturbation, the bogus disease "phimosis," epilepsy, and "nervous diseases." Shockingly, the 1970 edition of the country's leading urological textbook informed a whole generation of medical students that a long foreskin causes "rectal prolapse," malnutrition, epistaxis (nose bleed), convulsions, night terrors, chorea (muscle twitching), and epilepsy.[44] The highly respected author assured medical students that: "[P]arents . . . are usually ready to adopt measures which may avert masturbation. Circumcision is usually advised on these grounds."[45]

Circumcisers pushed the newly invented and extremely ludicrous myth that boys would be psychologically damaged if they were spared circumcision.[46] They repeated over and over again that circumcision was necessary for cleanliness and that no American child could ever be trusted to learn how to wash his own penis. Without mass circumcision, they insisted, women would be infected with cervical cancer and men would contract penile, prostate, and rectal cancer.

Many circumcision advocates even alleged that circumcision was necessary for military preparedness. Some hard-line military circumcisers, like Gerald N. Weiss, pounded out the falsehood that the intact penis required difficult daily washing, and that the lack of water during a military campaign would make hygiene impossible, leading to deadly infections.[47] It is hard to imagine that he actually believed this myth. Many American soldiers fighting in Vietnam were forcibly circumcised by military circumcisers under threat of court-martial. Some radical circumcisers, like Aaron J. Fink, ceaselessly shrieked the embarrassingly ridiculous myth that genitally intact soldiers would get sand under their foreskins and thereby be rendered unable to fight.[48] How could such a learned and well-educated physician actually believe this to be true? Yet, as ridiculous as this was, it was readily believed and is still repeated to this day. At the height of the Cold War, many Americans feared that war with the Soviet Union was inevitable, so it is easy to understand how the myth of military preparedness as an excuse for routine circumcision might have swayed some parents. Nevertheless, this is a perfect example of how circumcisers exploited, magnified, and exacerbated Cold War hysteria to frighten Americans into obediently remaining silent and unarmed when a circumciser came to cut their newborn sons.

THE DAWN OF INFORMED CONSENT

By the 1970s, doctors of good character and integrity realized that the situation was out of control. In 1971, the American Academy of Pediatrics Committee on Fetus and Newborn issued a warning to the nation that:

> *There are no valid medical indications for circumcision in the neonatal period.*[49]

Throughout the 1970s, Americans grew increasingly aware of the abuses of power rampant throughout the medical-industrial complex. They realized that their rights were routinely abused by forces operating within the health care system. Increasing numbers of Americans stood their ground and refused to allow circumcisers to touch their newborn children.

At the same time, parents initiated the grassroots movement for *informed consent.* This doctrine required hospitals honestly to tell patients about their condition, truthfully inform patients of their treatment choices, thoroughly explain the risks, disadvantages, and possible benefits of each treatment option, and obtain a legal signature before touching the patient. The doctrine of informed consent forbids doctors from withholding any information from patients and forbids them from using any degree of omission, coercion, or pressure to influence the patient to agree to any intervention. Ironically, the movement to stop hospital circumcisers from taking away parents' rights to protect their children from circumcision was spearheaded by Orthodox Jewish families. They were deeply offended that doctors had circumcised their babies without their knowledge or permission because this destroyed their plans to have their children ritually circumcised in a religious ceremony eight days after birth, as required by their branch of Judaism.[50] Hospitals were sued, and parents won.

A major ethical problem with newborn circumcision is that the person undergoing this medically unnecessary and contraindicated surgery is too young to understand what is happening to him, to consider his options, and to refuse the surgery. He is too young to defend himself against those who would take advantage of him. Reluctantly, spokesmen for the circumcision industry conceded that parents might give consent for their children by proxy. Obviously, these industry spokesmen have a glaring conflict of interest. Furthermore, they can hardly be considered ethicists. Their interest is promoting and profiting from circumcision rather than protecting people's rights. Ethically, no one has the right to provide proxy consent for medically unnecessary surgery. Only in the case of life-threatening emergencies is proxy consent valid.

Many unsuspecting parents expressed their intention to protect their sons from circumcision and refused to sign the consent form. I have heard many tales of nurses and doctors bullying such parents by coming into the mother's hospital room at all hours, demanding that the consent form be signed. In some instances, the hospital circumcised the baby first and then handed the mother the consent form for signature.

This illegal practice has resulted in a number of lawsuits, one example of which cost a hospital $1.4 million in June 2001.[51] In this case, the hospital kept the baby hidden from the mother, pretended that the baby was still intact, and demanded the signature on the consent form *after* the circumciser had executed the circumcision in a slipshod manner, permanently crippling the child. This case is rendered all the more tragic because the parents had decided long ago to protect their baby from circumcision and had expressly told the hospital that the baby was *not* to be circumcised.

THE RISE OF THE CIRCUMCISION INDUSTRY

Has money had anything to do with the persistence of circumcision? You decide.

Today, circumcisers charge between $121 to $300 per circumcision.[52] For physicians with busy metropolitan practices, 150 to 200 circumcisions a year can bring in as much as $60,000 extra through this one surgery alone. That is enough for a brand-new, four-door Mercedes sedan, annual membership fees at a country club, and several new pairs of Gucci loafers every year.

Nationwide, with 1.2 million healthy baby boys needlessly

being put under the circumciser's knife, circumcisers are collecting between $145 million and $360 million each year. Of course, this is just the amount of money that the circumciser takes home. When you add in all of the related "hidden" hospital and doctor charges resulting from the procedure, as well as the cost of hospitalization, legal fees, multimillion-dollar lawsuit settlements, and surgical reconstruction fees related to the complications, the cost of routine circumcision to insurers and parents in the United States is astronomically high.

One hidden factor that raises the cost of circumcision to the health care industry is the additional cost of the hospital stay for circumcision. Between 1990 and 1991, researchers discovered that the difference in hospital length of stay between newborn boys who leave the hospital genitally intact and those who end up being circumcised amounts to an annual cost between $234 million and $527 million *beyond* the charges for the procedure itself.[53]

To look at the big picture, HCIA-Sachs, a leading health care information company, reports that the total cost of an in-hospital nontherapeutic neonatal circumcision in the United States has risen from $1,154 in 1992 to $1,869 in 1999. This represents a cost increase of 62 percent. The total cost of all neonatal circumcisions performed in hospitals in the United States was reported to be $2.1 billion in 1999![54] In these times of increasingly scarce health care dollars, it is difficult to justify wasting all that money on a surgery that is unnecessary and contraindicated—a surgery that amputates part of the penis from someone who might have preferred that his penis be left alone if he had been given the dignity of a choice over his own body. Instead of being wasted on penile reduction surgery, imagine if that money were spent on a worthy and urgent cause like breast cancer research.

As you can see, circumcision is extremely profitable, forming a bread-and-butter income for the medical-industrial complex. Yet, this is hardly the end of the story. The aftermarket for human foreskins is where the real money is made. Parents should be wary of anyone who wants to cut off their baby's foreskin. Human foreskins are in great demand for any number of commercial enterprises, and the marketing of purloined baby foreskins is a multibillion-dollar-a-year industry. The human foreskin has been commodified without the permission or knowledge of the majority of Americans.

Pharmaceutical companies use foreskin in the manufacture of interferon and other drugs. Corporate researchers use human foreskins for a wide range of experiments, searching for new profit horizons. International biotech corporations are procuring cells from amputated foreskins and experimenting with artificial skin. Products like LifeCell Corporation's AlloDerm or Advanced Tissue Sciences' Dermagraft-TC, which sells for about $3,000 per square foot, are grown from the unique cells in infant foreskins and used as temporary wound coverings. One foreskin contains enough genetic material to grow 250,000 square feet of skin.

According to a report in *Forbes* magazine, the annual market for baby-penis-derived products could be $1 billion to $2 billion.[55] Advanced Tissue Sciences has sold about $1 million worth of cultured foreskin products to Procter & Gamble, Helene Curtis, and other such businesses for premarket testing. Advanced Tissue Sciences' foreskin-derived merchandise helped generate a $32 million stock offering in the beginning of 1992.

It is distressing to learn that biotechnology firms like Organogenesis have suspiciously received fast-track approval from the Food and Drug Administration for its foreskin-based Graftskin. American doctors, medicolegal experts, and bioethicists were denied the opportunity to request a full hearing and voice their concerns over the ethics of trafficking in and marketing human sex organs that have been harvested for this purpose without the permission or knowledge of the "donor."[56] In January 1998, when an FDA committee was formed to review Advanced Tissue Sciences' application for approval of its baby-foreskin-derived product, Dermagraft, they gave a respected human rights attorney only five minutes to speak to the committee in defense of Americans whose foreskins are cut off and marketed without consent or financial compensation. On May 26, 1998, the FDA hastily granted Organogenesis approval for what amounts to legalized plunder of our children's bodies.[57]

THE DECLINE OF ROUTINE CIRCUMCISION

Despite the economic pressure to continue and increase the scheme of mass involuntary circumcision, the rate of circumcision has declined in this country as a result of the combined efforts of enlightened doctors, nurses, and caring parents just like you. In 1975, the American Academy of Pediatrics had organized another Task Force Committee on Circumcision that issued an even stronger policy statement against circumcision that concluded:

> *There is no absolute medical indication for routine circumcision of the newborn. . . . A program of education leading to continuing good personal hygiene would offer all the advantages of routine circumcision without the attendant surgical risk. Therefore, circumcision of the male neonate cannot be considered an essential component of adequate total health care.*[58]

Insurance companies all over the nation welcomed this change and ceased paying for routine circumcision. The income and power base of circumcisers was now directly threatened. Furthermore, a series of high-profile lawsuits over circumcision disasters in which the entire penises of several babies were burned off and destroyed during "routine" circumcision generated very bad publicity for the circumcision industry.[59] One heartbreaking case that concluded in 1991 cost an Atlanta hospital $22.8 million.[60] Circumcision advocates reacted by engaging in damage control. A professionally orchestrated backlash against the expressed will of the American people was soon unleashed.

Coupled with the upsetting revelations that babies were being killed and crippled by routine circumcision, the old rationales for circumcision were losing their effectiveness. Unbiased doctors and researchers were proving that all the standard medical justifications for mass circumcision were imaginary and fraudulent.[61] To compensate for the loss of such long-lived excuses as the prevention of masturbation and epilepsy, circumcisers hastily sought to invent new justifications for an existing medical practice.

As I will explain in greater detail in the next chapter, Thomas E. Wiswell, in 1985, came up with the theory that circumcision reduced the rate of urinary tract infection.[62] This publication launched his career as one of the most vociferous advocates of mass circumcision this country has ever seen. In 1986, the mass circumcision extremist Aaron. J. Fink (1926–1994) invented the myth that circumcision prevented AIDS.[63] In 1993, circumcision militant Dr. Gerald N. Weiss seized upon this idea and launched the theory that the foreskin was afflicted with special cells that made it especially susceptible to HIV infection.[64] In 1973, a trio of circumcision fanatics—R. Dagher, Melvin L. Selzer, and Jack Lapides—felt so threatened by the popular movement away from circumcision that they actually published an article insinuating that anyone who disagreed with their agenda of mass circumcision was mentally ill.[65]

Many doctors naively accepted the new circumcision myths as if they were fact, never suspecting that the inventors of these myths had preexisting biases and conflicts of interest that should have raised doubts in anyone's mind about the motivations of these advocates and the soundness and genuineness of their "data." Consequently, few noticed when a handful of determined circumcision advocates began lobbying and pressuring the American Academy of Pediatrics in 1986 to reverse its policy on circumcision.[66]

Under the able leadership of Dr. George W. Kaplan, the chairman of the AAP Urology Section, the AAP resisted this pressure for three years. Sadly, though, after years of persistent barrage and infiltration, the AAP eventually caved in to pressure and organized a new Task Force on Circumcision. This time, the task force was instigated and chaired by Edgar J. Schoen, who was an advocate for mass circumcision.[67] Ethically, Schoen's bias should have excluded him from the committee. Not all the members of the new committee, however, abandoned their scientific and ethical principles in the face of the intense barrage of extremist intimidation aimed at them. Consequently, after intense debate and bickering, the circumciser-dominated task force in 1989 was able to issue a new statement that took into account Wiswell's urinary tract infection hypothesis. The statement tenuously suggested that "newborn circumcision has potential medical benefits and advantages as well as disadvantages and risks."[68] Nevertheless, the hard-line anti-foreskin ideology of the committee's chairman should make intelligent people question the scientific validity and ethical scope of the 1989 task force statement. Especially unprofessional is the fact that the task force statement ignored the large scientific literature documenting the unique anatomical, physiological, and erogenous benefits offered by the foreskin and intact penis.

One of the longest nails in the coffin of routine circumcision was the publication in 1996 of a landmark anatomical study of the innervation of the foreskin by a research team at the University of Manitoba. Led by Dr. John R. Taylor, the team described the structural and functional components of the foreskin and established its rich erogenous innervation and vascularization.[69]

After extensive review of the medical literature on circumcision, including Dr. Taylor's study, both the Australian College of Paediatrics and the Canadian Paediatric Society published policy statements on neonatal circumcision in 1996.[70] Both organizations recommended that circumcision of newborns should not be routinely performed, and both statements acknowledged that circumcision contravenes human rights.

Finally freed from domination by circumcisers, the AAP organized its most recent Task Force on Circumcision, under the responsible leadership of Dr. Carole M. Lannon, which released a revised statement on circumcision in 1999. Although imperfect in many ways, the new statement has undone most of the damage of the 1989 statement and admits that the alleged and, in my considered medical opinion, *imaginary* medical "benefits" are "*not* sufficient to recommend routine neonatal circumcision."[71] (Italics added.)

Despite the persistent efforts of circumcision extremists to reverse the trend, the rate of circumcision has been steadily declining in the United States. The latest report from the Centers for Disease Control and Prevention has revealed that circumcision rates have dropped at a remarkable speed.[72] Soon, circumcision will be a relic of the past. In the Western states of America, the circumcision rates dropped from 62 percent in 1980 to less than 37 percent in 1999. For the whole country, the rate has dropped from 67.8 percent in 1995 to 65.3 percent. The data show that the reason that the national rate has failed to fall as dramatically as it has in the Western states is because circumcisers have been targeting blacks and other minorities— groups that previously were less likely to be circumcised. As the rate of circumcision of white babies has fallen, the rate for black babies has risen.

Increasing numbers of concerned American doctors and nurses are lending their support to the movement to purge medical practice of circumcision. Professional organizations such as Doctors Opposing Circumcision and Nurses for the Rights of the Child have been empowering health care workers to help defend our babies from unnecessary surgical interference and educate parents about the anatomy, functions, normal development, and proper care of the normal human penis.

In the face of increasing popular rejection of routine circumcision and the increasing respect for the miracle that is the human body, I am confident that circumcision will soon be a thing of the past. The American people are now reclaiming their ancient heritage in preserving and honoring the human body as nature designed it.

Chapter 8

● ● ●

Are There Medical Benefits to Routine Circumcision?

I believe the time has come to acknowledge that the practice of routine neonatal circumcision rests on the absurd premise that the only mammal in creation born in a condition that requires immediate surgical correction is the human male. If the penile foreskin is not merely nonfunctional but a biological disadvantage so severe as to justify its immediate surgical ablation, then, surely, it might have atrophied by now.[1]

Thomas Szasz, M.D.

Would your son be healthier if part of his penis were cut off? Are there really any benefits to circumcision? If so, what could these benefits be? What possible benefits could be so important, overwhelming, and compelling that they could justify subjecting a child to desensitizing, denuding, and disfiguring penile reduction surgery without his permission or consent? Are these benefits important enough that you would be willing to put your child at significant risk of a serious surgical accident to his penis?

If you were to consult a standard medical textbook, published in the last five years, about the supposed medical benefits of infant circumcision, you would get one answer. If you looked at a textbook from thirty years ago, the answer would be different again. If you looked at a medical textbook from the 1950s, you would get a different answer still. Finally, if you looked at a textbook from the 1890s, you would find that the alleged medical benefits of circumcision are even more different.

As we've seen, in the 1960s and 1970s, when the campaign for systematic, compulsory circumcision was already institutionalized in most U.S. hospital complexes, circumcisers were still telling parents that routine circumcision was medically *necessary*—even mandatory!—to stop masturbation, convulsions, nervousness, night terrors, epilepsy, and other entrenched bits of quackery left over from the nineteenth century.[2] Consequently, most of the adult circumcised Americans alive today were circumcised for these ludicrous "medical" reasons rather than for any of the so-called medical benefits that are being peddled today. History, however, proves that even these new benefits will be seen as quackery by future generations of doctors.

The strange fact is that the promoters of infant circumcision keep changing the list of supposed "benefits." As soon as one "benefit" is disproved, they invent another one to take its place. There is no other surgery in all of medicine like this. Imagine if doctors were still trying to find justifications for other common nineteenth-century surgical horrors such as bloodletting, trepanning (drilling holes in the skull), clitoridectomy, castration, routine snipping of the frenulum that holds the tongue to the floor of the mouth, or amputation of the uvula. This is precisely the strange situation we are in with circumcision.

Circumcision is unique for the tremendous number of benefits that circumcisers have ascribed to it and for the intensity of the drive to come up with new rationale for an old compulsion.

This fact alone should put intelligent Americans like *you* on guard. When I was in school, I was taught that the more reasons offered to justify something, the less likely it is that any of them are true.

Some hard-line advocates of mass circumcision try to make circumcision seem more acceptable and noninvasive by drawing a false analogy between it and routine immunization. Circumcision and immunization cannot be equated because, unlike circumcision, immunization does not result in the loss, diminishment, desensitization, alteration, or change in the appearance or function of any body part. Every circumcision results in these irreversible changes. Additionally, immunization effectively prevents us from spreading highly infectious, communicable diseases that you cannot reasonably avoid through healthy lifestyle choices. Before immunization, these diseases caused terrible epidemics. Serious diseases such as smallpox, tuberculosis, and measles are spread just by casual, minimal contact or by breathing in the exhaled air of an infected person. The diseases of which circumcision is supposed to reduce the rate fail to meet this definition. They are all either noncommunicable or spread by unsafe sexual contact with infected partners. Any sensible American can avoid these diseases by making healthy lifestyle choices. Circumcision has never protected anyone from the negative health consequences of poor lifestyle choices. Finally, immunization is highly effective at preventing the spread of disease. Even using the questionable and flawed data created by circumcisers, circumcision is highly ineffective at reducing the rates of any disease. As you will see, the alleged differences in the rates of targeted disease between circumcised and genitally intact males is infinitesimal, barely reaching statistical significance and never reaching clinical significance.

In this chapter, I will examine the medical-sounding myths that prevail today. These are the issues that the 1999 American

Academy of Pediatrics Task Force on Circumcision examined and decided were too insignificant for them to recommend routine circumcision.[3] This is an important fact that parents are interested to learn. I find that parents are also very interested to learn that *all* of these so-called benefits were invented by a small band of well-positioned, vocal, and determined circumcised men whose animosity toward the foreskin was well established before they embarked on the highly questionable course of manufacturing data that appeared to support their agenda. These men display a glaring conflict of interest. Additionally, I will examine some of the myths that the AAP has debunked but which you may still hear today.

PENILE CANCER

Circumcision is hardly a logical way to prevent penile cancer. It would make just as much sense to amputate the breast from all young girls to prevent breast cancer. The myth that the foreskin causes penile cancer was largely invented in 1932 by Abraham L. Wolbarst.[4] As I pointed out in the previous chapter, Wolbarst was one of the twentieth century's most militant promoters of mass circumcision and one of the first to demand that newborn circumcision be made compulsory, allegedly to prevent penile cancer, but also for the prevention of epilepsy, convulsions, and masturbation.[5]

The myth was given a further push by New York urologist Abraham Ravich, who also invented the now debunked myths that the foreskin causes prostate cancer[6] and cervical cancer in women.[7] Even without any clinical data to support his wild theory, Ravich insisted that smegma—the harmless and beneficial penile lubricant—was a carcinogen. Amputation of the foreskin, he argued, removed the glands that produce smegma, thereby making a male immune to cancer.

Every modern attempt to prove that smegma causes cancer, however, has failed.[8] Smegma no more causes cancer of the penis than tears cause cancer of the eye. In her classic paper "How Smegma Serves the Penis," Dr. Joyce Wright revealed how important and useful this natural body secretion is.[9]

There are many scientific flaws with the penile cancer myth. First of all, normal body parts cannot cause cancer in other body parts. In the last few decades, scientists have learned that complex human diseases like cancer are almost certainly caused by a combination of environmental factors, behavioral factors, and, sometimes, defective genes. The normal, intact penis no more gives itself cancer than breasts give themselves breast cancer.

I find it fascinating that penile cancer is one of the rarest male cancers. This is probably because the intact penis has such a magnificent blood supply and highly evolved immune defenses. Penile cancer is also one of the most treatable forms of cancer if caught in the early stages of its long development. Urologist colleagues of mine have informed me that the reason *any* American men die of penile cancer at all is because these men usually wait *decades* after the first indications of cancer have appeared before seeking medical help. By then, it is too late. Thus, penile cancer is deadly only if men make poor health decisions.

Did you know that penile cancer is so rare that the government feels it unnecessary to keep statistics on it? Did you know that more American men contract and die of breast cancer than penile cancer? These are important facts that should put the whole matter into perspective.

The best estimate is that the United States, where the majority of adult males have been subjected to neonatal circumcision, has a rate of penile cancer of 1 or 2 in 100,000.[10] This is two to three times *higher* than the rate of penile cancer in non-circumcising, First World countries such as Denmark,[11] Finland,[12] and Japan.[13] Clearly, the myth that circumcision prevents penile cancer is false. Advocates of universal circumcision cannot counter these facts, so they ignore them and hope that you will never find out.

Who gets penile cancer? Scientific studies have proven that penile cancer is almost exclusively limited to elderly, poverty-stricken, uneducated men—usually minorities—with a history of poor hygiene, chronic smoking, alcoholism, repeated venereal infections, and promiscuity.[14] Objective studies prove that *smoking* is the single largest contributing factor in the production of penile cancer.[15] With a lifestyle as unhealthy as this, penile cancer is usually the least of these men's problems.

As the large generation of males targeted for newborn circumcision after World War II grows older, so the rate of penile cancer among circumcised elderly males increases in direct proportion. A 1993 study found that 79 percent of patients with penile intraepithelial neoplasia (a form of penile cancer) had been circumcised at birth or in early childhood.[16] A subsequent study found that 9.5 percent of twenty-five patients with penile intraepithelial neoplasia or carcinoma in situ (another form of penile cancer) had been circumcised at birth.[17] The circumcision status was unrecorded, however, in 16 percent of the patients. Another important study documented Bowenoid papulosis of the penis (an early stage of penile cancer) in eleven young males, ten of whom had been circumcised at birth.[18] These large-scale studies demonstrate that the total number of cases of penile cancer is hardly limited to intact males. Instead, they show that penile cancer is limited to poor, uneducated males with a lifetime of terrible hygiene.

A recent study from Los Angeles County indicates that, in addition to the risk factors mentioned above, a lifetime of chronic physical inactivity is also a prime risk factor for penile cancer.[19] This large-scale study found that "phimosis" was unassociated with carcinoma in situ and only mildly associated with invasive carcinoma. Additionally, the researchers discovered that when they adjusted circumcision for "phimosis" in their study, either by including it in the logistic regression or by limiting the analysis to men who never experienced "phimosis," the alleged "protective" effect of newborn circumcision essentially disappeared. The researchers, however, failed to define what they meant by "phimosis" and failed to explain how they measured it. Nonetheless, they found that circumcised males are particularly susceptible to clinical infections with sexually transmitted diseases, such as genital warts (HPV) and herpes. This is significant because genital warts are strongly associated with the development of penile cancer.

Even if circumcision did prevent penile cancer, this would hardly justify newborn circumcision. Penile cancer is just too rare. It would make more sense to subject newborn boys to routine removal of breast tissue. After all, breast cancer is far more common among men than penile cancer. Penile cancer is also highly treatable if caught in the early stages of the disease. Why should healthy boys have invasive surgery forced on them for a disease that almost none of them will ever get?

In any event, the studies show that circumcision is ineffective in preventing penile cancer. The best thing you can do as a parent is to teach your child to lead a moral, clean, and healthy life. Make education a high priority in your family. Teach your child the value of cleanliness. Teach your child to avoid smoking, drugs, and promiscuous, unprotected sex with anyone, especially infected partners.

I know that you were planning to do this anyway. Just by being a good parent, you have already done everything humanly possible to instill in your child the good habits that will provide him with a lifetime of protection from diseases of all kinds.

URINARY TRACT INFECTIONS

One of the latest scare tactics designed to implant, magnify, and exploit the fears of new parents and even doctors is the myth that circumcision prevents urinary tract infections in the first six months of life. The truth is that cutting off part of the penis is an unscientific way of preventing UTIs.

This myth is based on a controversial methodologically flawed "study" that was produced by an advocate of mass circumcision named Thomas E. Wiswell in 1985.[20] The scientific fact is that UTIs are exceedingly rare in boys. Girls get UTIs at far greater rates. Additionally, you will be very glad to know that UTIs are easily treated with antibiotics, and, more important, effortlessly and naturally prevented by breast-feeding,[21] proper hygiene, and a healthy diet.

Objective scientific studies have found that UTIs are almost exclusively limited to boys with urinary tract anomalies. This means that these boys were born with internal deformities along the urinary tract—the two tubes that run from the kidneys to the bladder and then exit the penis through a single tube called the urethra. Most of the time, males with these deformities enjoy perfectly normal lives, never knowing that something is unusual with their urinary tract. A urinary tract infection is often the first helpful clue to doctors that anomalies are present. X-rays can usually reveal whether these anomalies can be safely ignored or whether they will require surgery. The foreskin has nothing to do with this. Indeed, the early diagnosis of a UTI may be lifesaving, because any congenital problem can then be treated or corrected by appropriate urological surgery.

Most significantly, a Canadian study from 1998 proved the worthlessness of the 1985 study. Although it failed to control for race, breast-feeding, maternal urinary infection, urine collection method, diagnostic criteria for UTI, and family history of UTI, it nevertheless found that the UTI rate for intact infants was only 3.7 times higher than for circumcised babies.[22] In other words, the rate of UTI for intact and circumcised boys appeared to be 0.154 percent and 0.034 percent, respectively. This is only a *0.1258* percentage point difference. It is considered to be *statistically* significant, but it certainly cannot be considered to be *clinically* significant. In short, this study documented that 99.846 percent of genitally intact boys will never contract a UTI. Those who do develop a UTI should be treated just like doctors treat girls and circumcised boys—with antibiotics.

Finally, I would like to draw your attention to an important study on UTI that was presented at the annual meeting of the American Academy of Pediatrics in 1997. The authors found that:

> *Regardless of circumcision status, infants who present with their first UTI at 6 months or less are likely to have an underlying GU (genitourinary) abnormality. In the remaining patients with normal underlying anatomy and UTI we found as many circumcised infants as those who retained their foreskin.*[23]

This only confirms that circumcision is ineffective at protecting your baby from this rare and minor problem. Even if it somehow did, it is senseless to subject 195 randomly selected healthy babies to penile reduction surgery on the off chance that this *might* spare a single boy from an easily treatable UTI.

Can you imagine how your child would feel if you had to tell him that you allowed yourself to be talked into permitting a circumciser to amputate his foreskin to "protect" him from UTI—during his first six months of life—an extremely rare, yet easily treatable infection that he was never likely to get anyway?

Remember that the surest way of preventing UTI is to leave your baby's foreskin alone, breast-feed, keep your baby clean, and change his diapers whenever necessary. Mother and baby form a unit. The more you hold your baby and enjoy skin-to-skin contact, the more you will be protecting him from diseases of all kinds.

SEXUALLY TRANSMITTED DISEASES

Circumcision is powerless to prevent the spread of sexually transmitted diseases. The mistaken idea that circumcision prevents the acquisition and spread of STDs is an old myth from the nineteenth century that gained new impetus in the 1940s, through the determined efforts of urologist Eugene A. Hand.[24] At this time, there was a general panic in the medical profession over African-American soldiers spreading STDs.[25] It is important to remember that this was in the days before penicillin was cheaply and widely available. STDs were hard to treat and doctors had little understanding about how they were transmitted.

As with penile cancer, most American males with gonorrhea or syphilis were poor, uneducated, rural, lower class, sexually promiscuous, and usually of minority race. This category of American was less likely to be circumcised than middle-class white males who were born in private hospitals where compulsory newborn circumcision had been instituted.

Even so, large-scale studies of all kinds performed by objective researchers have found that circumcised men have higher rates of most major STDs than intact males. This is a shocking fact that circumcisers have tried to cover up.

A famous study on nongonococcal urethritis (NGU) concluded:

> *A case-control study of active duty soldiers showed that both Black and White circumcised subjects were 1.65 times as likely to have NGU as uncircumcised subjects.*[26]

The authors of another valuable 1994 study on the relationship between circumcision and STDs—especially the various types of gonorrhoea—concluded that:

> *Circumcision of men has no significant effect on the incidence of common STDs in this developed nation setting. . . . We determined no association between circumcision status and a history of NGU or gonorrhoea. In the case of gonorrhoea this may have been because this was uncommon in our population; the slight trend was for the presence of a foreskin to be "protective."*[27]

An exhaustive 1994 study on herpes simplex virus type 2 (HSV-2) concluded:

> *[W]e found no evidence of the presence of an intact foreskin being a risk factor for HSV-2 infection.*[28]

A classic 1993 study on genital warts, also known as human papilloma virus (HPV), came up with the unshakable conclusion that:

> *[U]ncircumcised men had a lower prevalence of genital warts than circumcised men. . . . [T]he presence of the*

foreskin may confer nonspecific protection of the proximal penis from acquisition of HPV infection.[29]

Dr. Robert Van Howe conducted the largest review of the scientific literature on STDs and circumcision ever published. His conclusions are startling:

> *[T]he medical literature does not support the theory that circumcision prevents STDs.*[30]

To confirm this, the National Health and Social Life Survey conducted at the University of Chicago, found:

> *First, circumcision status does not appear to lower the likelihood of contracting an STD. Rather, the opposite pattern holds. Circumcised men were slightly more likely to have had both a bacterial and a viral STD in their lifetime.*[31]

Circumcised males had higher rates of all bacterial and viral STDs. Circumcised males had higher rates of nongonococcal urethritis, herpes, and chlamydia—one of the most common STDs today. One must ask why circumcisers have been insisting that circumcision does prevent STDs and have been getting away with this bogus claim for so long.

The plain fact is that it is unimportant how much penis you have; what you do with it determines your risk for contracting STDs. Your sexual behavior and lifestyle choices affect your risk of disease rather than your circumcision status. After all, STDs are unable to fly through the air and infect innocent people. You have to work hard to get an STD. This category of disease is contracted as a result of poor decision making.

Neither circumcision nor intactness can affect your decision-making abilities. More important, neither circumcision nor genital intactness will save you from the consequences of poor decisions.

HIV/AIDS

Of all the charges leveled against the human foreskin, none is more frightening—*and none warrants closer scrutiny*—than the ongoing, well-publicized charge that it predisposes its possessor and his sexual partners to an early, slow, agonizing death—from infection with the AIDS virus.

Let us first reflect on the incontrovertible fact that the United States has the largest number of sexually active circumcised males and the highest rate of HIV and AIDS in the developed world. Clearly, circumcision is powerless to prevent AIDS. Where, then, did this myth come from?

As we have seen, this myth was invented in 1986 by California urologist Aaron J. Fink, a militant crusader for compulsory newborn circumcision. Fink spent his retirement years firing off angry letters to editors of medical journals, fighting for media airtime, engaging in backroom politics in the California Medical Association, and pushing a self-published manifesto—all for the promotion of mass involuntary circumcision of American males.

In an unexpected departure from its fastidiously high scientific standards, the *New England Journal of Medicine* actually published, without demanding any scientific substantiation, one of Fink's tirades against normal human anatomy in the form of a letter to the editor.[32]

Fink claimed that the keratinization, or callused thickening, of the glans of the circumcised male reduced the chance of HIV infection. Fink had no data to back up his claim. He just made it all up. Another prejudiced myth that Fink borrowed from Eugene A. Hand[33] and relentlessly pushed was that the foreskin is likely to tear or develop "micro-fissures" during sex, allowing HIV to enter the bloodstream. This ridiculous myth is repeated frequently by other circumcised circumcisers even today.[34] Needless to say, there is *no* scientific evidence to support this ludicrous myth. It is just another crude fiction. I find it highly ironic that it was invented and circulated by circumcised males who cannot know what sex is like with a normal and intact penis.

Even though Fink had no rational basis or evidence to support these notions, they were taken up with great vigor by several vocal circumcision crusaders. A flurry of studies—all of which were conducted in Africa, of all places, for highly suspect reasons that I will explain below—were whipped up in an attempt to prove Fink's idea and provide further excuses for the continuation of involuntary circumcision of newborn males in the United States. All of these African studies, however, have serious flaws, and none have been able to find anything more than a tiny fraction of a difference in HIV infection rates between genitally intact and circumcised Africans.

You see, the problem for circumcisers is that the United States has the highest percentage of sexually active circumcised males *and* the highest rate of HIV in the developed world.[35] In fact, the rate of HIV in the United States is higher than that of many Third World countries! The noncircumcising countries of Europe have the *lowest* rates of HIV in the entire world. Clearly, mass circumcision has failed to protect any Americans from AIDS. These facts are deeply embarrassing for anyone trying to pretend that circumcision has health benefits.

To prove that circumcision has no effect on HIV infection rates in First World nations such as the United States, a very important study conducted at the National Centre in HIV Epidemiology and Clinical Research and at the National Centre in HIV Social Research in Sydney, Australia, determined that the circumcision status of homosexual men infected with HIV by receptive or insertive unprotected anal intercourse was unimportant.[36] Genitally intact and circumcised Australian males who engaged in unprotected anal intercourse had equal rates of HIV infection. The research team also found that men who had seroconverted despite having avoided unprotected anal intercourse were also just as likely to be circumcised as genitally intact. Consequently, the foreskin is innocent of any role in HIV infection in homosexual, Western men. Other, more obvious sites, such as the anus and distal urethra, are the more likely locations of HIV infections.

Australia is a First World nation with a standard of living equal to that of the United States. Sharing a very similar culture, its population can logically be compared and equated to that of the United States. Africa is another story altogether. Since all of the "studies" being used to support the myth that circumcision prevents AIDS have been conducted in Africa, let us carefully examine these studies and determine why they are both flawed and irrelevant to the United States and, thus, to your child's health.

Studies from Africa

African countries have the highest rates of HIV and AIDS in the world. Also, African countries that have the highest rate of HIV also have high rates of circumcision. Nevertheless, the first wave of circumcision promotion consisted of geographical studies of Africa, which studied maps rather than living men. Using decades-old anthropological data, extrapolating HIV incidence rates, and employing complex statistical manipulations, a tiny association was made to appear between the African foreskin and HIV.[37]

Next came a number of observational studies suggesting an association between the foreskin and an increased risk of HIV infection in men, mostly in Kenya, who exhibited high-risk behaviors.[38] Who were these infected men? Promiscuous, illiterate, lower-class long-distance truck drivers who were frequent and habitual customers of HIV-infected prostitutes.

Does this sound like the lifestyle of the average middle-class American male? Should American males be surgically altered because of the poor decisions of promiscuous African truck drivers in Kenya?

The Flaws in These African Studies

One fundamental flaw in these African "studies" is that they fail to control for important variables. Many of these variables, including sexual, religious, and hygienic practices, as well as economic status, appear to be linked to tribal affiliation, which, in turn, is strongly correlated with circumcision status.[39] Many of the circumcised Africans in these studies are Muslims. Islam requires stricter sexual and hygienic practices. This alone could account for the minuscule difference in rates between circumcised African Muslims and genitally intact African non-Muslims. The fact that these important cultural factors play a major role in behavior and HIV susceptibility make it incorrect and *irresponsible* to place blame for HIV's spread on normal penile anatomy.

Dry Sex

There is another important factor in the African AIDS crisis that American circumcisers have deliberately ignored in their studies: *dry sex.* Dry sex is a pervasive practice in sub-Saharan

Africa. Studies from Zimbabwe, Zaire, Malawi, Zambia, the Central African Republic, and South Africa have documented the prevalence of the bizarre practice of drying and/or tightening the vagina by smearing it with dried leaves, sand, dirt, cornmeal, or powders to absorb the vaginal lubrication.[40] Africans supposedly believe that this practice makes sex more interesting.

Dry sex, however, dramatically increases HIV infection risk. It causes various problems with condom usage, is associated with an increased rate of STDs in men, and an increased rate of HIV among women. Dry sex is associated with increased lesions, lacerations, peeling of the vagina, chlamydial infection, and epithelial trauma in both male and female. In this way, it creates an easy portal of entry for HIV.

Because of this increased risk, dry sex is an obvious confounding factor in any study of HIV and circumcision in sub-Saharan Africa. Yet, all of the approximately forty existing studies promoting the idea that circumcision prevents AIDS have ignored this factor.

Irresponsible Sexual Behavior While Afflicted with Genital Ulcer Disease

Yet another factor that is ignored in antiforeskin studies is rampant sexual activity while suffering from genital ulcer disease (GUD), a type of venereal disease. Genital ulcer disease, endemic in parts of Africa, is a very strong risk factor for HIV infection.[41] These lesions may provide an entry point for the HIV virus. One study discovered that South African Zulu men with bleeding genital ulcers often continue to have sexual intercourse with women, including prostitutes.[42] Another reported on the prevalence of GUD in prostitutes in Kenya, noting that many prostitutes continue to work despite having the disease.[43] Therefore, the presence of GUD becomes a significant confounding factor in any study that attempts to make meaningful conclusions about the relationship between circumcision status and HIV susceptibility.

Female Circumcision

The African practice of female circumcision is yet another contributing factor to the spread of HIV that has been ignored by circumcisers.[44] Male circumcision is always found where female circumcision is practiced. Because the circumcised vulva may be sewn shut, the male sexual partners of circumcised females often resort to anal intercourse. This is a proven risk for HIV transmission.

Circumcised Males Aren't Immune to the Negative Consequences of Promiscuity!

In some of these African studies, a certain percentage of the circumcised African males who engaged in promiscuous and unsafe sex with HIV-infected prostitutes or wives may genuinely have been HIV negative at the time they were interviewed for the study. One Ugandan study, published in the year 2000, looked at 415 couples in which one partner was HIV positive. It claimed to find that over the course of ten months, fifty circumcised African males avoided becoming infected with HIV and forty genitally intact African males did contract HIV.[45]

Does this mean that circumcision prevents HIV? No. As leading AIDS expert Dr. Laurence Peiperl points out: This conclusion is illogical, as the small sample size and the short duration of the study and follow-up allow for the significant and probably inevitable possibility that these circumcised subjects would eventually contract HIV if they continued to have sex with HIV-infected wives and prostitutes.[46] Also, the fact that over one third of the circumcised men in this study were HIV positive on entry demonstrates that circumcised Africans are being infected with HIV at enormous rates.

Another factor is religion. The 2000 Ugandan study found that Ugandan males who were circumcised in childhood claimed to have lower rates of HIV than Ugandan males circumcised in adulthood. What does this mean? This study failed to control for religion, but a 1999 study by the same authors, using the same Ugandan population, confirmed that 79 percent of the circumcised males were Muslims. Also, most of the HIV-positive males circumcised in childhood were Muslims and most of the HIV-positive men circumcised in adulthood were non-Muslims.[47] Since Muslims are proven to be less likely to engage in risky, promiscuous sex, this alone could account for the tiny difference in HIV infection rates found in the 2000 study.

This study tells us that a promiscuous circumcised African male who has risky sex with HIV-infected prostitutes may be temporarily HIV negative on the date that an American researcher interviews him, but *nothing* will stop him from becoming HIV positive the next day, the next week, or the next year if he continues his irresponsible behavior.

Irresponsible high-risk sex with HIV-infected partners will eventually result in disease whether you are circumcised or genitally intact.

Even if these African studies had some validity—and I seriously doubt they do, given the proven bias and conflict of interest of their authors—it is impossible to apply them to the United States or other developed countries.

The imposition of mass circumcision on the United States is unscientific and a threat to the integrity of the medical profession. Any true scientist knows that you can compare only like with like. The health statistics of the United States can be compared only with those of countries with similar standards of living, like the countries of Europe.

Why Do Noncircumcising European Countries Have Dramatically Lower Rates of AIDS than the United States?

One answer may be the protective immunological functions of the foreskin. The foreskin contains glands that produce lysozyme[48]—an enzyme secreted in human bodily fluids that acts to destroy bacteria, fungi, and other infectious agents. Bacteria are capable of producing lesions through which the HIV virus can enter the body. Lysozyme has long been known to destroy the cell walls of bacteria. Scientists have discovered that lysozyme is an effective agent for killing HIV directly in vitro.[49]

What Do Leading American Medical Societies Say?

After reviewing all the literature on AIDS and circumcision, the Task Force on Circumcision of the American Academy of Pediatrics concluded that:

> *Behavioral factors appear to be far more important risk factors in the acquisition of HIV infection than circumcision status.*[50]

The Council on Scientific Affairs of the American Medical Association has also examined the issue. In their report, the council stated:

> *Behavioral factors are far more important risk factors for acquisition of HIV and other sexually transmissible diseases than circumcision status, and circumcision cannot*

be responsibly viewed as "protecting" against such infections.[51]

What Can You Do to Protect Your Child from AIDS?

This is simple: Teach your child that it is *suicide* to engage in promiscuous, risky, unsafe, and unprotected sex. Teach your child the values of personal responsibility, self-control, dignity, self-worth, and a committed monogamous relationship. Cutting off part of your child's penis cannot protect him from the consequences of bad decisions and is no substitute for good parenting.

Make your home loving and supportive. Be generous with your love and forgiveness. Love your children with your whole heart, but also be a guide, teacher, and role model. If you create a loving, affectionate, secure, and supportive family environment for your children, they will be more likely to grow up with the vital sense of self-worth and dignity that will preserve them from making poor lifestyle choices. As a parent, it is your responsibility to convey these values.

HYGIENE

The myth that circumcision makes the penis cleaner is very common. Nevertheless, it is false. I find it strange that the people who insist that this myth is true are usually circumcised doctors who can have no idea what they are talking about, never having had the benefit of personal experience with a normal penis. It is a fact that the normal penis with its foreskin intact is perfectly clean. It stays clean all by itself without any extra effort.

Even if circumcision somehow did make the remaining

parts of the penis cleaner, this would never be a sufficient reason for cutting the foreskin off. The mouth would be cleaner if all the teeth were removed in childhood. Without teeth, we would never have to brush them. The hands are among the dirtiest parts of the body. If we routinely cut babies' hands off, we would never have to bother washing them.

If you take this argument to its extreme, where would we stop cutting? These arguments, as you can see, are unscientific. We live in a modern world of soap and fresh running water. Surgical amputation of body parts is hardly a rational substitute for soap and water.

Besides, the foreskin keeps itself clean. In this respect, the foreskin is analogous to the eyelid. Just as the eyelid keeps the eye clean, safe, moist, warm, and protected, so the foreskin keeps the glans clean, safe, moist, warm, and protected. Cutting off the foreskin is like cutting off the eyelids. Would your eyes be cleaner if your eyelids were cut off? You are intelligent enough to know the answer to this.

The normal penis with its foreskin intact is free of any need for special care. It is free of the need for special washing. In fact, the best thing for your child is just to leave his foreskin alone. Never try to retract your child's foreskin. Never try to wash underneath it. Just leave it alone. It is self-cleaning, just like the eyes.

Mothers used to be advised to retract the foreskin and wash beneath it. Some misguided doctors still give out this very harmful advice. This is very bad advice indeed! When the foreskin becomes fully retractable, usually by the end of puberty, your son can gently and easily retract it and rinse his glans with warm water while he is in the shower. It takes only a second.

I should indicate here that it is my considered medical opinion that circumcision actually makes the penis dirtier. This fact was confirmed by a study recently published in the *British Journal of Urology.*[52] The explanation is simple.

For at least a week after circumcision, the baby is left with a large open wound that is in almost constant contact with urine and feces—hardly a hygienic advantage. Additionally, throughout life the circumcised penis is open and exposed to dirt and contaminants of all kinds. The wrinkles and folds that often form around the circumcision scar frequently harbor dirt and germs.

Thanks to the foreskin, the intact penis is protected from dirt and contamination. While this important protective function is extremely useful while the baby is in diapers, the foreskin provides a lifetime of protection to the glans and urinary opening. At all ages, the foreskin keeps the glans safe, healthy, and clean.

What Is Smegma?

Some people are concerned with smegma. There is no reason for concern about smegma in the foreskin any more than there is reason for concern about the presence of tears in the eyes. Both are supposed to be there. Both tears and smegma serve useful functions. Females, in fact, produce smegma in far greater quantities than males. Do you hear doctors advocating female circumcision in order to keep the vagina clean?

Smegma is clean. As we learned in Chapter 1, smegma is a natural secretion that keeps the glans penis clean, moist, soft, lubricated, and free of harmful bacteria. It is a thin, white, creamy secretion. It is usually found in minute quantities in the groove behind the glans—the coronal sulcus. It is supposed to be there just as tears are supposed to be in the eyes to moisten and clean them.

A famous study of 9,200 Danish schoolboys found that visible smegma was present in only 5 percent of boys, the incidence increasing from 1 percent in the six- to seven-year-old boys, to 8 percent in the sixteen- to seventeen-year-old boys. It is during puberty that smegma increases, as would be expected. The author noted:

> *Production of smegma increases from the age of about 12–13 years. Neither this nor the hygiene of the prepuce present any problems.*[53]

How would you ever explain to your child why you permitted a circumciser to cut off the end of his penis? Would you tell the truth and say: "Son, we had you circumcised because we thought you would be too stupid to learn how to wash yourself"?

It is a good thing for parents to be concerned with cleanliness. It is good for parents to lovingly encourage their children to enjoy the sensation of being clean. Make daily baths or showers a joyous ritual in your home. Teaching children the joys of bathing is one of the honored responsibilities of parenthood.

I suppose that some people used to think that circumcision would free them from having to bother with cleaning their child's penis. They were sadly misinformed on many levels because the intact penis is free of any need for extra care. Just leave it alone, and it will take care of itself.

PHIMOSIS

There is no such thing as phimosis. There is especially no such thing as phimosis in children. This is a bogus "condition" or "disease," largely invented by nineteenth-century quacks looking for an easy way to hustle gullible people out of their money.

Today, circumcisers make a diagnosis of "phimosis" because

they are ignorant of the facts of normal penile development and because that is what they were taught to do in medical school. Since many insurance companies refuse to pay for *routine* circumcision, doctors and hospitals fraudulently swindle reimbursement out of insurance companies by claiming that newborns are being circumcised as a cure for the disease "phimosis" rather than simply as a matter of hospital routine.[54] This is medical fraud, pure and simple, and *you* are paying for it through increased insurance premiums.

Circumcisers define phimosis either as a foreskin that is "too long," a foreskin with a small preputial orifice that protects the glans from premature exposure, or a foreskin that is attached to the glans. These are all normal developmental stages of the baby's penis. Pretending that these normal stages of penile development are a deformity is like pretending that a newborn's lack of teeth is a deformity of the face and mouth.

Too Long?

There is no such thing as a foreskin that is "too long." Most of the medical texts that use this definition define "excessive length" or "redundancy" as any foreskin that completely covers the glans. This is unscientific quackery. It represents a size limit that almost no boy could ever meet, thereby giving circumcisers license to cut. Foreskins come in all sizes and lengths. Some boys are generously endowed with impressively long foreskins and others have foreskins that barely cover the glans. All are normal and healthy.

Too Narrow?

The remaining two definitions for phimosis are equally ludicrous. You see, a child's foreskin is supposed to be nonretractable. The orifice is supposed to be small. This is a beautifully engineered feature that protects the immature glans from premature exposure. It keeps the glans and the urinary opening clean, warm, moist, and protected from danger. As a boy grows and matures, the orifice will gradually become more elastic. Studies show that, by the end of puberty, almost all boys will have a foreskin whose preputial orifice is elastic enough to allow the glans to protrude fully.[55] Erections also play a helpful part in increasing the diameter of the preputial orifice.

Attached?

Similarly, the attachment of the foreskin to the glans is normal and highly protective in babyhood and childhood. Nearly all boys are born with the foreskin still fused to the glans. Over time, the glans and foreskin slowly separate and develop their own surfaces. This is a natural process of penile development. Like the elasticity of the preputial orifice, the natural separation of the glans and foreskin takes almost two decades. It is during puberty that hormones speed up this process. Erections also play a part in separating the foreskin from the glans.

Many circumcised doctors in the United States are unable to understand—or *refuse* to understand—these biological facts. They continue to call these natural developmental stages of the penis a "condition" or "disease" called "phimosis" or "penile problems." They are wrong. Imagine if doctors insisted that young girls were diseased because their breasts are smaller than the breasts of adult women! Imagine if doctors insisted that babies were suffering from a brain disorder because they were unable to talk at birth!

Just like the rest of his body, the penis of a child is immature at birth. Maturation takes decades. It is only when puberty has been completed that the penis will be fully developed.

What about BXO?

In England, the highly respected pediatric surgeon A. M. K. Rickwood has been instrumental in educating the medical profession on these important points of human anatomy. He has published numerous scientific papers calling for the unscientific use of the word "phimosis" to be abandoned.[56] He would like it to be used exclusively to describe a penis that is afflicted with a clinically verifiable case of the extremely rare disease balanitis xerotica obliterans. This disease is so rare that scientists are unaware of what causes it. It presents as a hard, white plaque on the skin of the penis. It can cause the normally supple and elastic skin of the penis to become hard and inelastic. There is no mistaking BXO. It is instantly recognizable by trained doctors.

BXO, however, is easily cured by steroid creams applied directly to the affected area.[57] Surgical removal of the affected parts is almost never necessary. When surgery is necessary, it is perfectly possible to remove the BXO without resorting to circumcision.[58] This allows the patient to keep a normal-looking and fully functional foreskin.

What if an Adult Still Has a Nonretractable Foreskin?

A small fraction of adult males have foreskins that resist full retraction. If this is due to attachment of the glans to the foreskin, and if the man wants them to be separated, these attachments can easily be gently separated in the doctor's office with local anesthesia. Circumcision is hardly necessary.

If the adult foreskin resists retraction because the diameter of the preputial orifice is narrow, this can also be remedied *if* the man wants it to be remedied. French researchers have found that a simple regime of daily manual massage and stretching of the foreskin can greatly increase the diameter of the adult preputial orifice.[59] Penile skin is highly elastic and responsive to stretching. These exercises are simple, free, and effective.

It is interesting to note, however, that many males with non-retractable foreskins are happy just the way they are. They enjoy the security, the streamlined look, and the feel of a foreskin that always covers the glans. Genital cleanliness is just as easy with a nonretractable foreskin. It may even enhance sexual activity. Since the foreskin is double-layered, the upper layer can slide over the inner layer, thereby stimulating the glans and, simultaneously, being stimulated by the glans. A foreskin that remains in place during erection is always in a state of readiness for this natural and efficient mechanical mode of penile stimulation.

CERVICAL CANCER

The myth that male circumcision prevents cervical cancer in females was disproved long ago. Still, one hears it repeated by ignorant doctors. As I mentioned earlier, this myth was largely invented in 1951 by the determined circumciser Abraham Ravich.[60] In 1954, it was given an additional push by the New York physician Ernest L. Wynder (1922–1999).[61]

Wynder and especially Ravich did everything they could to popularize this myth in medical journals, newspapers, and popular magazines.[62] The hypothetical association between the foreskin and cervical cancer seemed to give females the impression that they had a personal stake where routine male circumcision was concerned. It tricked them into imagining that sex was dangerous and unhealthy. The cervical cancer myth drove a wedge between men and women. Unsurprisingly, then, some females, influenced by misinformation from biased doctors, have actually supported routine circumcision on this illegitimate basis, as demonstrated in popular writings on the subject.

Wynder and his associates, however, based their assumption of the circumcision status of the male partners of women with cervical cancer on the results of a questionnaire filled out by their women patients. In 1958, however, a similar study found that a large percentage of men were wrong about their circumcision status.[63] Men who were circumcised thought that they were intact. Men who were intact thought that they were circumcised.

In a follow-up study, published in 1960, Wynder reevaluated and retracted the results of his 1954 study[64] because erroneous patient reporting had been a source of considerable statistical error. Wynder found that 3 percent of female patients in Los Angeles were ignorant of the circumcision status of their husbands. In New York, 38 percent of women were unaware of the circumcision status of their husbands. Twenty-four percent of two hundred male patients were unable to correctly state their circumcision status. In another paper, Wynder again conceded that his 1954 findings were invalid.[65]

Unsurprisingly, Wynder's follow-up studies were ignored, while circumcision advocates continued to promote his invalidated 1954 study. Still, many responsible researchers who conducted studies in the United States, Europe, and elsewhere found that there was no association between cervical cancer and the circumcision status of male sexual partners.[66] Researchers did find, however, that the true risk factors for cervical cancer are early age at first intercourse, early age of first episode of genital warts, multiple sexual partners, previous history of sexually transmitted diseases, multiple births, and smoking.

No matter how one interprets the motivations behind misstatements of circumcision advocates, mentioning cancer of the penis or cervix in connection with circumcision needs to be recognized for what it is—a deliberate scare tactic calculated to mislead.

Women, if you want to protect yourselves and one another from cervical cancer, circumcising your sons is futile. You will have to take personal responsibility for your own life. Avoid smoking and promiscuous sex. It's that simple.

DOING IT NOW TO AVOID DOING IT LATER

Many mothers have come to me in anguish over this issue. They want to spare their baby the pain and discomfort of circumcision, but they have heard a frightening tale of some neighbor's son who *had* to be circumcised because of an infection or some other problem with the foreskin. A mother will usually say to me: "I don't want to put my son through that, so maybe he should be circumcised now."

As you can see, this is an example of how irrational fears cloud our judgment. An intelligent and compassionate mother can be so afraid that there could be a *chance* that her son *might* need a circumcision someday that she is willing to put him through the ordeal of penile surgery now even though he is healthy. Does that make sense?

I suppose that some mothers are able to entertain such an illogical view because they have been misinformed that circumcision is painful for older children but not for babies. It is a scientific fact that the pain and trauma of circumcision is far more intense for a baby than it is for an older child or adult. After all, an older child would be given anesthesia and postoperative pain relief. Babies are almost never provided with any form of pain relief. Even if they are, however, the surgery and postoperative period are painful for the baby. The younger the baby, the more intensely he feels the pain.

A mother may also be aware that circumcision in older children can cause severe psychological and emotional traumas. As

Dr. Benjamin Spock and other various psychologists have been warning parents for decades, many older boys who undergo circumcision experience emotional damage that lasts a lifetime.[67] The shock of losing part of his penis can be overwhelmingly devastating for a child. Many never recover. Many never forgive their parents.

Still, the misguided assumption is that circumcision in the newborn period has little effect upon the mind. This we know to be untrue as well. Study after study shows that newborn circumcision has a profoundly detrimental effect upon the brain. We often fail to recognize these problems because they have become nearly universal. They seem like normal male behavior in a society where the vast majority of adult males were circumcised at birth.

Nevertheless, the other blatantly irrational element of this all too common reason for newborn circumcision is the myth that some other child *had* to be circumcised. In my many decades of pediatric practice, I have never had a patient who had to be circumcised. Problems with the foreskin are extremely rare, but when they arise, I can always determine what is needed to fix them without surgery. If a boy gets an infection in his foreskin, I treat it just as I would an infection of any other part of the body: I use antibiotics. They always work. If parents would just follow the simple rule of never touching or attempting to retract their child's foreskin, infections are unlikely ever to occur. Clearly, a doctor who insists that a boy must be circumcised just because of an infection is wrong. He should be told so, and he should be reported to the hospital administration.

Many doctors will mistakenly tell parents that a child will have to be circumcised if the foreskin cannot be fully retracted after age three. This, as you have learned, is completely wrong and utterly unscientific. The foreskin and the glans form a unified whole. They are supposed to be attached to each other dur-

ing childhood. It takes nearly two decades for the process of separation to be complete. The process of separation is gradual, slow,
and gentle. It is usually complete by the end of puberty. There is
never any medical need to rush this process of maturation.

So you see, if you ever hear about some boy who *had* to be
circumcised, you can be certain that this boy was circumcised
unnecessarily under false pretenses. This is a very sad example of
medical ignorance and medical fraud. The real tragedy is that an
innocent child has been made to suffer the consequences of
adult fears, irrationalities, and ignorance.

After investigating these topics, it should be clear that circumcisers never invented these myths to advance the cause of
medicine. They have been attempting to manufacture a web of
medical-sounding justifications to rob us of our constitutional
freedoms to privacy and sovereignty over our own lives and
bodies.

After years of examining this issue, it is my view that the so-
called benefits of circumcision are little more than the elaborate
and confusing smoke screen that circumcisers use to hide their
true goal of invading, interfering, overregulating, controlling,
and curtailing our private lives. The more benefits they can invent, and the more convincing they seem, the more confident
circumcisers feel that they can get away with marring the body,
wounding the spirit, and censoring the life of another human
being who is helpless to stop them. By robbing him of his foreskin, circumcisers are literally severing a male from a means of
perceiving, experiencing, sharing, and enjoying his existence.

I think that nearly all parents want to do what's best for their
children. Even the most confident-appearing parents have self-
doubts about the wisdom of their child-raising methods. All
parents make mistakes, even with the best of intentions. We are
all human. Having a child for the first time can bring up a lot
of fears in young parents. They want to do the right thing. They

want guidance from experts. Sadly, circumcisers have shown that they never have our children's best interests at heart. They have exploited the fears of parents and tricked them into a surgery that no rational parent would agree to if given all the facts.

Let us banish fear from child care. Let us embrace our human heritage and respect the principles of human dignity. Let us trust in nature's beautiful and elegant design for the human body. Let us trust in the wisdom of nature and several million years of evolutionary refinement of the human body. Let us protect our children from unnecessary surgery and, once again, make parenting the joyous privilege that it is supposed to be.

Chapter Nine

● ● ●

Common Nonmedical Excuses for Routine Circumcision

> Defending circumcision requires minimizing or dismissing the harm and producing overstated medical claims about protection from future harm. The ongoing denial requires the acceptance of false beliefs and misunderstanding of facts. These psychological factors affect professionals, members of religious groups and parents involved in the practice. Cultural conformity is a major force perpetuating non-religious, and to a greater degree, religious circumcision. The avoidance of guilt and the reluctance to acknowledge the mistake and all that it implies help to explain the tenacity with which the practice is defended.[1]
>
> Ronald Goldman, Ph.D.

When I talk with parents about circumcision, I usually find that they are rarely concerned with the medical myths. Their anxieties are almost always related to nonmedical issues. In fact, I suspect that most of the parents who let a circumciser cut off the end of their baby's penis have done so because they were persuaded almost exclusively by nonmedical issues. What are these nonmedical issues? What nonmedical reasons could be so compelling that they could sway intelligent and compassionate parents to submit their healthy child to penile reduction surgery?

It turns out that these anxieties are generally related to issues of conformity.[2] This is strange because America was founded on the principles of individuality. Conformity should be the last thing that Americans are worried about, and yet, this is the most effective tactic that circumcisers have ever devised to sway parents. You see, most parents cannot be counted as circumcision fanatics. They are just looking for advice on a difficult topic. They are easy prey for someone with an agenda.

I am sure that somewhere, some parents may be real believers in circumcision, that is, lay people who have thought about the issues and have then consciously ignored the scientific and ethical facts and, instead, have forced themselves to accept the antiforeskin ideology. They constitute a tiny fraction of the parents who pay lip service to the medical myths and hand their babies over to a circumciser. The rest of the American people, however, allow their babies to be circumcised for no other reason than because they think that other parents are doing this. Rarely have they really made up their own minds. They are just following the crowd. They believe what they have been told to believe. They believe whatever they *think* the people around them believe.

With many parents today, it is much less a matter of really believing that circumcision is medically necessary as it is about believing what they *perceive* to be fashionable in their community. This perception most often comes from false assumptions. A middle-class circumcised father today may know that he is circumcised without really understanding what happened to him and how his life might have been different if he had been allowed to keep his whole penis. In reviewing his childhood, he may recall that other little boys—his brothers perhaps—were circumcised too. A mother may know that her husband is circumcised. She may recall that her brothers were circumcised. Although most parents have probably seen only a very small number of penises throughout their entire lives, they will, nevertheless, automatically assume that all males are supposed to be circumcised.

Certainly, boys born in the 1970s and 1980s, when the rate of newborn circumcision in the United States exploded to over 90 percent in some parts of the country, would have had very few opportunities to see a normal penis. Many males born in this era have no idea that they were circumcised. No one has ever told them that part of their penis was actually cut off. Many refuse to believe it when they are told. They think that they were born this way. One circumcised young man once told me that the first time he saw a normal intact penis on another boy in his high school locker room, he thought that he was looking at a penis that had been surgically altered in some strange way. When he learned that *he* was the one with a penis that had been surgically altered, he was shocked and horrified.

As I was saying, most parents assume that all boys are circumcised because the few penises that they have seen were circumcised. But this very common assumption is incorrect. Parents are basing their assumption on a situation that may have prevailed twenty or thirty years ago when they were children. They seem to be unaware that the circumcision rates were never really that high across the whole country and that they have dropped dramatically.

Another reason that common parental assumptions are incorrect is that parents are unaware of what goes on outside the borders of our country, in the advanced parts of the world. American parents are generally surprised to learn that newborn circumcision is unheard of in the Christian countries of Europe. Danish or Swiss parents, for example, would no more allow a circumciser to cut off part of their son's penis than they would allow a witch doctor to knock out one of their child's teeth or mark his face with tribal scars.

The most important thing that some parents have forgotten is that it is illogical to submit a child to surgery just because some other child may have had the same surgery. If every child on your street had his gallbladder removed, would you have your baby's gallbladder removed?

LOOKING LIKE DADDY?

One of the biggest anxieties that sometimes get in the way of parents' healthy instinct to protect their baby from harmful disturbances is the issue of a baby's looking like his father. I can assure you that circumcising a baby cannot make him look like his circumcised father, nor does it create a "bond" between the father and son. Bonds are created by the expression of love rather than by cutting the penis. A little boy's love and respect for his father has nothing to do with the father's penis. A little boy just wants his father to love him, guide him, and spend time with him.

The strange thing about this idea is that even the most intelligent and thoughtful fathers can become fixated on it. I think you will agree that it is very unhealthy and highly inappropriate for a father to be fixated on his son's penis. The idea of subjecting a baby to an operation on his little penis just because his father was subjected to the same operation is quite illogical. What if the father had a tonsillectomy? Would it be right to have the baby tonsillectomized so that he matches his father? What if the father were missing a finger? Would it be right to amputate a finger from the baby so that he matches his father?

I suspect that some of the anxiety that a few fathers have is rooted in competition and male rivalry. I was once counseling a pregnant couple about circumcision. I explained that the fore-skin serves many functions, that it is a normal part of the body, and that it has a wide range of sexual sensations and functions. The circumcised father turned to me and replied coldly: "I understand all this, but I don't see any reason why my son should have any more sensitivity than I do." His brutal rivalry toward his unborn son so shocked the mother that she was even more determined to protect her son from this man's baser instincts and cowardly approach to parenthood. Never have I seen a wife so disappointed and disillusioned with a husband.

It is very sad that the issue of circumcision, in some instances, can bring out the worst in fathers. We need to do everything we can to revive the old-fashioned American conception of fatherhood. A good father will want the best for his son. A good father will want to be generous toward his son rather than jealous and competitive. A good father will want his son to be more successful than he. A good father will want his son to have more opportunities than he did.

I think that we can all agree that it is inappropriate to circumcise a baby because his circumcised father might suffer from anxiety over the fact that his newborn son's penis looks different from his own. Cutting the baby's penis cannot solve the circumcised father's underlying problem that he may feel inadequate. He may be plagued by fears that others will think something is wrong with his penis. It would be best if mothers and family members encouraged fathers to be proud of their sons instead of being jealous or competitive toward them.

I find that most fathers who were born during the days of the post–World War II era phenomenon of mass circumcision are very interested to learn that the foreskin is an integral part of the penis. Rational fathers are also keenly interested to learn that circumcision results in the loss of at least 50 percent of the skin the penis, much of which, in most infants and children, extends well beyond the glans. Sometimes, the foreskin represents over half the length of the penis. I hardly think that any normal, mentally balanced male could remain indifferent about circumcision when he realizes that it shortens and desensitizes the penis. It is my experience that when the average father learns this information, he is usually eager to protect his newborn son from circumcision. He takes great pride in the fact that he is safeguarding his son's natural birthright. Most fathers want the best for their sons. They just need accurate information.

It would be best if parents remembered that it is senseless to operate on a healthy baby. We can justify performing operations in the neonatal period in response to genuine diseases, injuries, or deformities, but neonatal circumcision is never performed in response to a genuine medical problem. It is a surgery that, illogically, is performed on a perfectly healthy body part. This is unreasonable, as you will agree.

Each child is a unique gift, and that uniqueness should be cherished. The idea that a boy will be disturbed if his penis is different from his father's was invented to manipulate people into letting doctors circumcise their children. It has no basis in medical fact. There are no published reports of an intact boy being jealous when he realized that part of his father's penis had been cut off. When intact boys with circumcised fathers express their feelings on the matter, they consistently report their immense relief and gratitude that they were spared penile surgery. They also express sympathy for the suffering their dads experienced as infants when they were circumcised.

LOOKING LIKE OTHER BOYS

Another common excuse that I hear all the time is that boys should be circumcised if other boys in their family, neighborhood, or school are circumcised. This is hardly a legitimate reason for subjecting a child to penile surgery.

In many cases, it represents a psychological projection onto the child of parental anxieties over conformity. Your son hardly needs to be circumcised just because some relative or some boy down the street is circumcised. Besides, chances today are that the boys in your neighborhood are genitally intact.

The most insidious part of this myth is that it assumes that you will be a bad parent. It implies that you will be unable to instill in your child a sense of self-worth. Let's say that your boy does discover that some boy down the street was circumcised. Why would you assume that your boy will be envious and will want to have the end of his own penis cut off? Naturally, when you think about it, you realize that you would never assume such a thing. But circumcisers have brainwashed a great many parents into believing this.

I have every confidence that you will do everything you can to be a great parent. I know that you will do your best to teach your child self-respect. There is no doubt in my mind that you will teach your child to honor his body. It would be best if you were also to teach your child to *respect* rather than *envy* other children. If some little boy down the street was unfortunate enough to be circumcised, remind your child how lucky he is to be blessed with a whole body. After all, your child has something precious. The child down the street had that thing taken away from him. Now, who should be envious of whom?

THE LOCKER ROOM MYTH

One of the excuses that circumcisers sometimes use to try to persuade parents to agree to the circumcision of their children is that a genitally intact boy will be teased in the high school locker room by his circumcised peers. There is no evidence to support this ludicrous myth. It is clearly just another insidious persuasion tactic designed to rob American males of sovereignty over their own bodies. Nevertheless, in these times, I find it very hard to believe that any boy would dare make a public comment about the penis of another boy.

Even if some parents were tricked into believing this myth, I can assure you that it is ridiculous. Parental anxieties that a genitally intact son may be teased by his peers in school are illegitimate grounds for overriding the individual's right to bodily integrity. Parents who have been led to believe this myth are usually just projecting onto their children their own remembered traumas suffered as a result of obsolete institutionalized humiliations, such as compulsory communal showering in school—a practice that has largely been abandoned in American schools today, even though parents may be unaware of this change.

Even if compulsory showering is still a part of your child's high school physical education class, so what? There is no reason to imagine that your child, with his intact body, would be envious of a boy whose foreskin had been amputated. Children quickly realize that each body is unique and different. Sometimes parents need to be reminded of this. We must remind ourselves of the simple fact that all children know: Everyone is unique and different in his own way.

Furthermore, let us remember that it is impossible to predict how a boy will feel about his own penis. If he has been raised in a good home and has been raised to be strong-willed, responsible, and confident, he will prefer his intact penis as it is. He will be very glad and enormously relieved that no one cut off part of his penis. What sort of child would want part of his penis cut off just because some other child suffered such a fate? After all, your son, with his intact penis, is the normal one.

Imagine if a bitter one-legged child teased your child for having two legs? Would your child take such teasing seriously? You know in your heart that he would be above such things. In any event, when your son reaches adulthood, he is free to have himself circumcised if that is his wish. A child circumcised at birth has been denied all options and choices over his own body in this regard.

Also, teasing is hardly a medical problem. Likewise, circumcision for this reason has no medical value, and, if performed, necessarily violates the human rights of the child. Similarly, there is no guarantee that a genitally intact boy will be teased. Also, there is no guarantee that your child would even care if some disturbed child did tease him. The child who suffers from the compulsion to tease will always find something to tease another child about. In any event, teasing is more appropriately handled by discipline and psychological counseling for the teaser rather than by ill-conceived attempts at preemptive surgery for the potential victim of teasing.

Even if you still find it difficult to let go of the anxieties planted in your mind by propaganda from circumcisers, you will be interested to learn that this excuse is even less valid than ever before. Thankfully, more and more American parents are rejecting the un-American practice of circumcision. The rate of circumcision is dropping rapidly. Chances are, most boys in your child's neighborhood and school are being protected from circumcision.

WHAT IF OUR SON ASKS QUESTIONS?

Some circumcised fathers worry that they will be unable to find the right words to say when their son asks why his penis looks different from his father's penis. Children are curious, which is a wonderful thing about them. Curiosity enables their intellects to grow. It stimulates brain development. It is best to encourage and applaud a young boy's natural curiosity about the world.

Inevitably, a boy who was permitted the dignity of keeping his penis intact may discover that his circumcised father's penis looks different. He may well ask the reason for this difference. When this question arises, parents can answer it easily. They need only say: "Son, when Daddy was born, some doctors thought that it was a good idea to cut off the foreskin. Now we know that this operation is unnecessary. That's why you have all of your penis, just the way it is supposed to be."

Some intact boys may find out that some of their friends were circumcised. They may ask why. You can answer this question very easily as well. Just say: "Son, you have all of your penis because we protected you from circumcision. Circumcision is unnecessary. Your friend is circumcised because his parents were unaware that circumcision is a bad idea. They may have received some incorrect information from their doctor."

As we have seen, the most powerfully persuasive reasons for circumcision tend to be social and religious rather than medical. Even circumcisers are strong believers in the social reasons and often use the medical excuses only as convenient window dressing to hide their real motivations. Doctors have taken an oath to heal the sick. They have never taken an oath to perpetuate social customs or blood rites. That is hardly their job.

None of these social rationalizations are sufficient justification for subjecting an innocent and healthy person to an amputative surgery without his permission. After all, he is the one who must spend the rest of his life with the circumcised penis. It seems incredibly unfair that a child should be circumcised because his parents are uninformed and unable to free themselves from their own conditioning. Children are human beings who deserve the same respect and consideration that we would accord any other valued member of our family. It is time that we realize that these so-called social reasons for circumcision are just clever pressure tactics devised by circumcisers. Let us free our children from these un-American attempts to compromise our freedoms and subvert our culture.

Chapter 10

• ● ●

Most Common Reasons Given for Postneonatal Circumcision:
How to Protect Your Genitally Intact Son from Unnecessary Penile Surgery

> Whatever is done to stop the terrible practice of circumcision will be of tremendous importance. There is no rational medical reason to support it. . . . It is high time that such a barbaric practice comes to an end.[1]
>
> Frederick Leboyer, M.D.

Increasing numbers of American parents today are protecting their sons from routine circumcision at birth, but as their boys grow up, they often find themselves at odds with doctors who cling to old-fashioned opinions and hospital routines. I often receive telephone calls from distraught parents who say that a doctor insists that their little boy needs to be circumcised because something is supposedly wrong with his penis. When they bring their son into my office, I almost always find that there is nothing wrong at all. On the rarest of occasions, there might be a slight redness, but this can be quickly cleared up with an antibiotic cream. In all my years of practice, I have never had a patient who had to be circumcised for medical reasons.

When a doctor advises that your son be circumcised, it's usually because he or she is unfamiliar with the intact penis, misinformed about the true indications for surgical amputation of the foreskin, unaware of the functions and normal development of the foreskin, and uncomfortable with the movement away from routine circumcision. In many cases, the doctor himself is circumcised. Consequently, the circumcised condition of his own penis as well as the usual psychological ego defense mechanisms may cloud his judgment. Some doctors are also unaware of the medical literature showing that circumcision during childhood can psychologically traumatize boys to an alarming degree. Some boys, circumcised during childhood, never really recover from the painful shock that part of their penis was amputated and that they are now walking around with part of their penis missing.

Finally, a doctor who recommends that your son be circumcised may have such a poor understanding of medical ethics that he fails to realize that it is unethical and inappropriate for him to surgically impose on your son—or on anyone, for that matter—his artificial, unnatural, culturally influenced, and limited conception of what a penis should look like. He may fail to understand that it is your son's penis and that, consequently, only your son has the right to make decisions about it. You see, despite the commonly heard objection that circumcision is no big deal, circumcision is, in fact, a big deal. It permanently affects the appearance and functions of the penis. As we have seen in the earlier chapters of this book, it destroys a remarkable and very useful body part. Circumcision is also a big deal, quite obviously, because of the intense determination some people have to impose it on others. Should your son be circumcised just to satisfy the psychological compulsions of another person?

I believe that parents ought to be made aware of the fact that many doctors can be psychologically challenged by the sight of an intact boy. They may see problems with the penis that are nonexistent. They may try to convince you that the natural penis is somehow difficult to care for. They may cite "studies" and "statistics" that appear to support circumcision. Probably, the only problem you will encounter with the foreskin of your intact boy is that someone will *think* that he has a problem.

The foreskin is a perfectly normal part of the human body, and it has very definite purposes, as do all body parts, even if we are unable to readily recognize them. You will be glad to learn that there is never any need to worry about your son's intact penis.

WHAT TO SAY WHEN THE DOCTOR RECOMMENDS THAT YOUR SON'S PENIS BE CUT

Below is a summary of some of the things that doctors have said to parents of young boys in an attempt to convince them to agree to circumcision. After each incorrect statement, I will give you the medical facts. This will help you understand that your doctor is ignorant of the anatomy, functions, development, and proper care of the normal, intact penis. This will also help you protect your precious child from unnecessary penile surgery. If you ever find yourself in a situation where a doctor suggests that your child should be circumcised, the best thing that you can say is simply: "Please, leave it alone."

"Your son's foreskin should be cut off in order to facilitate hygiene."
The truth is that the natural and complete penis with its fore-skin intact is self-cleaning. It is free of any special care require-ments. The very best thing is just to leave it alone. Circumcised doctors are often unaware of this. You may have to tell them yourself.

If a doctor ever makes such a comment to you, be sympa-thetic, but be firm. You are a lionness defending her cub. Re-mind your doctor that it is illogical to cut off body parts under the illusion that this makes the body cleaner. We would never amputate the labia of the female to improve feminine hygiene. We would never pull out our fingernails to improve hand hy-giene. We would never pull all the teeth to improve oral hy-giene. Therefore, no sensible person would amputate part of the penis under the misguided notion that this would improve gen-ital hygiene. Just leave the foreskin alone. It will take care of it-self. Trust in the wisdom of God's design for the body.

"Your son's foreskin is too tight. It doesn't retract. He needs to be circumcised."
The fact of the matter is that "tightness" of the foreskin is a safety mechanism that protects the glans and urethra from di-rect exposure to contaminants and germs. The "tight" foreskin also keeps the boy's glans warm, clean, and moist. As long as your son can urinate, he is perfectly normal. There is no age by which a child's foreskin must be retractable.

Be on your guard. Never let a doctor or anyone try to retract your child's foreskin. Optimal hygiene of the penis demands that the foreskin of infants and children be left alone. Premature retraction may tear the skin of the penis open, causing your child extreme pain. There is no legitimate medical justification for retraction. The child's discomfort is proof of that.

"Your teenage son's foreskin is too tight. It doesn't retract. He needs to be circumcised."

The simple anatomical fact of the matter is that sexual activity and erections are part of the natural process by which the lips of the foreskin become looser and the opening of the foreskin becomes wider. Circumcision is an illogical, irrational, and misguided approach to this situation. If a teenager would like to speed up the process of expansion, he can easily do so with simple stretching exercises.

The skin of the penis is noted for its great elasticity and for its ability to stretch and remain stretched. For twenty minutes, three times a day (or more if he prefers) the young man can grasp the lips of his foreskin with the fingers and thumb and pull it out, away from his body. Additionally, with clean hands, he can stretch open the foreskin opening, holding it stretched for as long as it is comfortable.

Eventually, with a little bit of patience and discipline, these exercises will result in a foreskin that everts and reverts over the glans with quickness and ease. Of course, it should be pointed out that there is no real anatomical need for the foreskin to evert and revert during sexual activity. Many males are glad that the lips of their foreskin stay securely closed under most circumstances so that the foreskin remains safely over the glans. It is a matter of personal choice. This is not a medical issue—this is a private issue that each male should be allowed to decide for himself.

"Your son's foreskin is 'adhered' to the glans. It must be amputated."

Again, the attachment of the foreskin and glans is nature's way of protecting the undeveloped glans from premature exposure. Detachment is a normal physiological process that can take up to two decades to complete. By the end of puberty, the foreskin will have detached from the glans because hormones that are produced in great quantities at puberty help with the process. There is no age by which a child's foreskin must be fully separated from the glans.

Some misguided doctors might suggest that the "adhesions" between the foreskin and glans should be broken so that your son can retract his foreskin. This misguided procedure is called synechotomy. To perform it, the doctor pushes a blunt metal probe under the foreskin and forcibly strips it from the glans. It's as painful and traumatic as having a metal probe stuck under your fingernail to pull it off. It will also cause bleeding and may result in infection and scarring of the inner lining of the foreskin and the glans. The wounds that are created by this forced separation can fuse together, causing true adhesions.

There is no medical justification for this procedure because the foreskin is supposed to be attached to the glans during childhood. If any doctor suggests this procedure for your son, firmly refuse, stating, "Just leave it alone!"

"Your son's foreskin is getting tighter. It no longer retracts. Something is wrong. He will have to be circumcised."
The simple truth is that, sometimes, in childhood, a previously retractable foreskin will become resistant to retraction for reasons that are unrelated to impending puberty. In these cases, the opening of the foreskin may looked chapped and sting when your son urinates. This is hardly an indication for surgery any more than chapped lips. This is just the foreskin doing its job. If the foreskin were missing, the glans and urinary opening would be chapped instead.

Chapping is most often caused by overly chlorinated swimming pools, harsh soap, bubble baths, or a diet that is too high in sugar, all of which destroy the natural balance of skin bacteria and should be avoided if chapping occurs. The foreskin becomes resistant to retraction until a natural and healthy bacterial balance is reestablished. You can aid healing by having your son apply a little barrier cream or some ointment to the opening of the foreskin. Live culture yogurt or just some pure acidophilus culture (which can be purchased from a health food store) can be taken internally and also applied to the foreskin several times a day to assist healing, and should be given any time a child is taking antibiotics.

"Your son's foreskin is red, inflamed, itching, and uncomfortable. It has an infection and needs to be cut off."
Sometimes the tip of the foreskin does become reddened. During the diaper-wearing years, this is just diaper rash. When normal skin bacteria and feces react with urine, they produce ammonia, which burns the skin and causes inflammation and discomfort. If the foreskin were amputated, the inflammation would be on the glans itself and affect the urinary meatus and enter the urethra.

When the foreskin becomes reddened, it is just doing its job of protecting the glans and urinary opening. Circumcision will have no effect on diaper rash. Amputating the foreskin would only ensure that the diaper rash will spread to the unprotected glans and urinary opening—a far more serious threat to your baby's health and comfort. If you should notice redness on your baby's sex organs, change your baby's diapers more frequently, and use a barrier cream until the rash clears.

Harsh bath soaps can also cause inflammation of the skin. Use only the gentlest and purest of soaps on your child's tender skin. Resist the temptation to give your child bubble baths, because these are harmful to the skin as well.

Foreskin infections are extremely rare, but if they occur, one of the many simple treatment options is antibiotic ointment along with bacterial replacement therapy (acidophilus culture).

A sensible doctor would never amputate a body part because of a simple infection. Most infections of the foreskin are actually caused by washing the foreskin with soap.[2] Leave the foreskin alone and remember that it is free of any need for special washing. If you do this, your child will be free of infections.

"Your son is always pulling on his foreskin. He should be circumcised."

I can assure you that, whether circumcised or genitally intact, all little boys touch and pull on their penis. It is perfectly normal. Intact boys pull on the foreskin because it is there to pull on. Circumcised boys pull on the glans because that is all they have to pull on.

Little boys sometimes will adjust the position of their penis in their underpants. They will also sometimes explore the interior of the foreskin with their fingers—a perfectly normal curiosity and nothing to worry about. It is important for parents to cultivate an enlightened and tender congeniality about such matters, otherwise they risk transferring unhealthy attitudes to their children.

Sometimes a boy will pull on his foreskin because it itches. All parts of the body itch occasionally. Even a circumcised boy has to scratch his penis from time to time. Just as it is unnecessary to worry every time your child scratches his knee, so it is unnecessary to worry when he scratches his penis. If the itch is caused by dry skin, then have your son avoid using soap on his penis. Treat the foreskin just as you would any other part of the body.

If the real fear is of masturbation, calmly remind yourself of this one simple and natural fact: All children will explore their bodies, including their genitals. While parents during the 1800s feared masturbation as a cause of disease, we now know that this fear is irrational and that masturbation is harmless and normal.

Touching their genitals gives children a pleasant feeling and relaxes them. Classic anatomical studies demonstrate that the foreskin is the most pleasurably sensitive part of the penis.[3] You can congratulate yourself for having protected your child from a surgical amputation that would have permanently denied him normal sensations.

"Your son's foreskin is too long. It should be cut off."

Any doctor who would say this is sending out a disturbingly irrational and unscientific message. It may be typical for some males—even male doctors—to be jealous of males with bigger genital endowments, but it is unacceptable and unethical for anyone to pretend that there is a legitimate medical justification for surgically reducing the size of another male's penis. We are dealing here with an unfortunate example of male rivalry rather than with medicine.

The anatomical fact that you should bear in mind is that there is tremendous variation in foreskin length. In some boys, the foreskin represents over half the length of the penis. In others, it barely reaches the end of the glans. All variations are normal. The foreskin is never "just extra skin" or "redundant." It is all there for a reason.

"Your child should be circumcised now because it will hurt more if it has to be done later, or worse, when he is an adult."

This mistaken notion is based on fear and on ignorance.

Circumcision is extremely traumatic for a young child. Knowing this, some mothers have accepted the misguided rationale that it is better to get the operation over with in infancy rather than risk the *remote possibility* that the child might require a circumcision later on.

This excuse is tragically wrong and has resulted in a very serious crisis in American medical practice. It is based on the false idea that infants and young children are unable to feel pain. Babies can see, hear, taste, smell, and feel. In fact, babies feel pain more acutely than adults, and the younger the baby, the more acutely the pain is felt.[4] The suffering of a baby undergoing circumcision is far greater than that suffered by an older child or adult.

If an older child or adult ever needed to be circumcised, he would be given anesthesia and postoperative pain relief. Doctors almost never give babies either of these.[5] The only reason doctors get away with circumcising babies without anesthesia is because the baby is defenseless and cannot protect himself. His screams of pain, terror, and agony are ignored or dismissed as unimportant. In any event, this all too common excuse is merely a scare tactic, one with tragic consequences for any baby forced to endure a surgical amputation without the benefit of anesthesia.

"Since your son is having anesthesia for another operation, we'll just go ahead and circumcise him."

Please be warned. Most parents are never told that their son is in danger of being circumcised during a tonsillectomy, or a hernia repair operation, an appendectomy, or a surgery for an undescended testicle. It would never occur to them.

If your child is going into the hospital for any reason, be certain that you tell the physician, surgeon, and nurse that under *no circumstances* is your child to be circumcised. Write: "No Circumcision or Foreskin Retraction!" on the consent form too.

If your child is circumcised against your wishes anyway, remember that you have legal recourse. Surgeons have *no* right to operate without express informed consent. Many parents have successfully sued doctors for needlessly, mercilessly, and autocratically circumcising their children.

Even the foreskins of adults can be very tempting to surgeons. A new mother told me that her eighty-three-year-old grandfather had recently fallen and broken his hip. When he awoke from the hip surgery, he discovered to his horror that he had been involuntarily circumcised. The surgeons never informed him that they might circumcise him. If they had, he would certainly have refused to consent to such a senseless violation. The grandfather suffered from a deep sense of loss and betrayal. To make matters worse, the severe pain in his penis made his recovery from the hip surgery much more difficult. We should all deplore and fight against this increasingly common hospital practice of circumcising the elderly—or anyone who cannot express themselves well—without their permission and without any legitimate medical indication.

That grandfather has a strong legal case against the doctors who did this to him, as was proven by a recent court case. In 1995, a genitally intact man underwent heart surgery at Earl K. Long Medical Center in Baton Rouge, Louisiana.[6] He woke up from the heart surgery and discovered that the surgeons had circumcised him without his consent, permission, or knowledge.

Caught redhanded, the surgeons pretended that the circumcision was a necessary part of the bypass surgery. No one fell for this flimsy cover-up. The victim successfully sued for medical battery and medical malpractice. No matter how much money he collects for his injury and betrayal, he will never have the foreskin of his penis back.

Some hospitals seem to have a policy of circumcising any genitally intact male who comes through their doors for any reason. As a matter of fact, a nurse from a hospital in New Orleans told me that her hospital had an unwritten policy of circumcising any African-American male of any age who came into the hospital for any reason. This sort of "racial profiling" or "gender profiling" is deeply disturbing and should be stopped.

"*Your son has cysts under his foreskin. He needs to be circumcised.*"

Such a remark is evidence of unacceptable ignorance of the normal development of the penis and foreskin. During the period when the foreskin is undergoing the slow process of detaching itself from the glans, smegma may collect into small pockets of white "pearls." These are hardly cysts.

Some doctors mistakenly think that the smegma under the foreskin is an infection, even though it is white rather than red, is cold to the touch, and is painless. As the foreskin proceeds with detachment, the body will do its job, and these pearls will pass out of the foreskin all by themselves. These collected pockets of cells are nothing to worry about. They are simply an indication that the natural process of detachment is occurring.

"*Your son has a urinary tract infection and needs to be circumcised to prevent it from happening again.*"

The mistaken idea that circumcision is a legitimate cure for a urinary tract infection is a medical fad that will soon pass. Medical research proves that UTIs are most often caused by internal congenital deformities of the urinary tract.[7] Amputating the foreskin cannot correct these internal deformities.

If your son gets a UTI, treat him the same as you would your daughter: Have the doctor prescribe the appropriate antibiotics; reduce the amount of refined white sugar in your son's diet; increase his intake of vitamin C; serve him cranberry juice on a daily basis. These are the time-tested treatments that work.

"*Your son sprays when he urinates. Circumcision will correct this.*"

Again, this remark is based on ignorance of the normal development of the penis. In almost every intact boy, the urine stream flows out of the urinary opening in the glans and through the foreskin in a neat stream. During the process of penile growth and development, some boys go through a period where the urine stream is diffused. Undoubtedly, many of these boys take great delight in this phase, while mothers, understandably, find it less amusing.

If your boy has entered a spraying phase, simply instruct him to retract his foreskin enough to expose the meatus when he urinates. He will soon outgrow this phase.

"Your son's foreskin balloons when he urinates. He needs to be circumcised or else he will suffer kidney damage."
The simple medical fact is that ballooning of the foreskin during urination is a normal and temporary condition in some boys. It results in no discomfort and is usually a source of great delight for little boys.

Ballooning comes as a surprise only to those adults who have no experience with this phase of penile development. Ballooning disappears as the opening of the foreskin increases in diameter. It requires no treatment.

"Your son caught his foreskin in the zipper of his trousers; we will have to cut it off."
A recommendation like this is both illogical and unethical. A zipper entrapment can cause discomfort and a little bleeding, and it is true that there have been rare cases where a boy has accidentally caught part of the skin of his penis in the zipper of his trousers,[8] but circumcision is unnecessary to remedy this situation. After all, would you cut off the glans of a circumcised child if his glans got caught in the zipper?

By cutting across the bottom of the zipper with scissors, the zipper can easily be opened to release the penile tissue. A little mineral oil will also help release the trapped skin.[9] Any lacerations in the skin can then be closed with either sutures or surgical tape, depending on the severity of the situation.

The proper standard of care in this situation is to minimize and repair the injury rather than make it worse by cutting off the foreskin and creating a larger and more painful surgical wound.

"Your son has 'phimosis.' He needs to be circumcised to correct this problem."

As we saw in Chapter 8, "phimosis" is often used as a bogus diagnosis when a doctor refuses to understand that the child's foreskin is supposed to be long, narrow, attached to the glans, and resistant to retraction. Some doctors are prescribing steroid creams for "phimosis," but this is unnecessary in children, since the foreskin is supposed to be safely attached to the glans in young boys. The naturally released hormones of puberty will help the foreskin become retractable at the appropriate time.

In adults who still have a foreskin that is attached to the glans or a foreskin with such a narrow opening that the glans cannot easily pass through it, steroid creams are a conservative therapy. This "therapy," however, need be employed only if the adult wants a foreskin that fully retracts. Many males prefer a foreskin that remains securely over the glans. It is purely a matter of personal choice, one that only each male can decide for himself.

"Your son has paraphimosis and must be circumcised to prevent it from happening again."

The simple fact is that circumcision is an inappropriate treatment for paraphimosis. It would be like amputating the foot to cure a twisted ankle. Paraphimosis is a rare dislocation of the foreskin. It is caused by the foreskin being prematurely retracted and becoming stuck behind the glans. Because of the pain involved in dislocating the foreskin like this, children rarely do it to themselves. Most often, it is misguided adults inappropriately trying to retract the child's foreskin prematurely. Please, just leave your child's foreskin alone.

The dislocation can most often be corrected by applying firm but gentle pressure on the glans with the thumbs, as if you were pushing a cork into a bottle. If you are unable to correct this yourself, you must seek medical attention immediately.

To reduce the swelling, doctors may apply ice to the penis or inject the foreskin with hyaluronidase.[10] Doctors in Britain have also reported good results from packing the penis in granulated sugar.[11] Sometimes, the swollen tissue may have to be gently punctured with a needle to withdraw the fluid that builds up in the trapped foreskin.[12]

Beware of doctors who want to perform a "dorsal slit." This is a mutilating operation that slits the foreskin lengthwise in half. It results in a strange, upside-down tuliplike foreskin and renders the foreskin useless in performing its protective functions. There is no reason to perform a dorsal slit. All the noninvasive methods outlined above are proven to be effective.

While writing this book, I received an anxious telephone call from a mother in North Carolina. Her six-year-old son had fully retracted his foreskin, causing it to get stuck behind the glans. The child did this because an ignorant doctor, who incorrectly thought that the boy's foreskin should be fully retractable, had ordered him to do this regularly. Neither the mother, the father, nor the doctors at the local emergency room could bring the swollen foreskin back over the glans where it belongs. With a conference call, I was easily able to instruct the mother in the very simple technique of gently squeezing the spongelike glans until it was small enough to allow the foreskin to return to its forward position over it. The boy's penis was back to normal in seconds. Both he and his parents were greatly relieved. With just a little knowledge, we were able to save the boy from the unnecessary and inappropriate circumcision that the ignorant and misguided emergency room physician was recommending and eager to perform. If you ever find yourself in a situation like this, remember that it is extremely important to deal only with physicians who value the foreskin, understand how it works, and know how to deal with any of the rare problems that may arise. A physician who recommends circumcision for penile problems should be avoided. He may be a wonderful doctor, a friend, or a respected figure in your community, but if he recommends circumcision, he is ignorantly providing your son with the worst possible care.

Let me repeat: Paraphimosis is almost always caused by inappropriate and misguided attempts by adults to retract the child's foreskin prematurely. There is no reason to retract a child's foreskin. Just leave it alone.

"Your son has BXO and will have to be circumcised."

Again, medical science has shown that circumcision is an illogical and extreme approach to this situation. Some doctors equate phimosis with an extremely rare skin disorder called balanitis xerotica obliterans, which is also called lichen sclerosus et atrophicus (LSA). BXO can appear anywhere on the body, but if this disorder affects the foreskin, it may turn the opening of the foreskin white, hardened, fibrous, and make retraction difficult. BXO is usually painless and progresses very slowly. Many times, it goes away by itself. To an experienced dermatologist, there is no mistaking BXO, but a diagnosis must be confirmed by a biopsy.

The good news is that BXO can almost always be successfully cured with steroid creams,[13] carbon dioxide laser treatment,[14] or even antibiotics.[15] Surgery should be considered only after every other treatment option has failed. Even then, circumcision is rarely necessary. Foreskin-sparing surgeries can remove the affected tissues and leave the boy with a normal-looking, functional foreskin.[16] Just as we would never amputate the labia of females with BXO or the glans of circumcised boys with BXO, it is logical that we should never consider amputating the foreskin of intact boys with BXO without first employing all of the conservative treatments that have proven their efficacy.

The intact penis needs no special care. Let your boy take care of it himself, and, when he's old enough, he will enjoy taking care of his own body. After all, it's his business. Just relax and avoid worrying about your son's intact penis. Remind yourself that the foreskin is a normal and natural part of the body. If European boys grow up healthy and unconcerned with their foreskins, so can your son.

Chapter Eleven

●●●

The Care of Your Son's Intact Penis

The worst foreskin problem most intact males ever have is that someone thinks they have a problem.[1]

John A. Erickson

Every newborn infant is special. It is amazing that the newborn baby is born *intact,* with eyes that see, ears that hear, a nose that smells, and skin that feels. The healthy newborn infant needs to be loved, to be nursed, to be held, to be talked to, to be touched, and to be protected.

Our beautiful babies need never experience agonizing pain. It is always best to protect our babies from such experiences. Our babies need never have part of their healthy bodies surgically amputated. After all, our babies are born perfect. They are made in God's image. No desert superstition, antiquated religious blood rite, or social custom is more important than the absolute right to bodily integrity.

An ancient ignorance has made the care of the newborn's penis seem quite complicated when, in fact, it is *very* simple.

"Just leave it alone" is the welcome commandment to all parents and health workers that should be heard around the world.

As we've seen, the foreskin has many functions. It keeps the glans of the penis warm, clean, moist, and sensitive. It protects against infection, and it keeps the urinary meatus safe from invasion by external contaminants. It is one of the means by which a baby perceives, experiences, shares, and enjoys his existence.

Repeating the advice of the American Academy of Pediatrics' 1984 brochure on the care of the foreskin is good advice to all parents, to all nurses, doctors, and health care workers: "Just leave it alone!"[2]

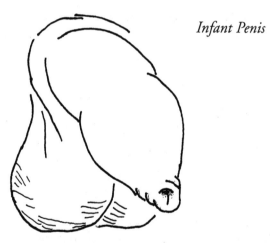

Infant Penis

Adapted from illustration
by Shaun Mather.

FORESKIN RETRACTION

During the first few years of a male's life, the inside fold of his foreskin is attached to his glans, very much the way the eyelids of a newborn kitten are sealed closed. The tissue that connects these two surfaces dissolves naturally over time—a process that should never be hurried.

The foreskin becomes retractable when its inside fold separates from the glans and its opening widens. This usually happens by age eighteen. Even if the glans and foreskin separate by themselves in infancy, the foreskin may still be unready for retraction because the opening of a baby's foreskin may be only large enough to permit the passage of urine. This is normal, protective, and necessary.

The first and only person to retract a child's foreskin should be the child himself.

A very young boy usually pulls his foreskin outward. This is normal and natural and no cause for concern. It is harmless and pleasurable. Once a boy discovers that his foreskin is retractable (a wondrous discovery for an intact child), he can easily learn to care for it himself.

WASHING THE FORESKIN

When the older boy is old enough to bathe himself, he can wash his penis when he washes the rest of himself. Simple instructions may be helpful.

1. Gently slip your foreskin back (only if it is fully retractable).
2. Rinse your glans and the inside fold of your foreskin with warm water.
3. Pat it dry if you like.
4. Slip your foreskin forward, back in place over the glans.

At puberty, you can let your son know that with hormonal activity comes new responsibility, including genital hygiene. He will find that keeping the penis clean is easy. It takes only a second. If you feel uncomfortable talking about genital hygiene, hand this book to your son and let him read it for himself.

WHAT CAUSES MY SON'S FORESKIN TO BE RED?

Sometimes the tip of the foreskin becomes reddened. This indicates the foreskin is doing its job of protecting the glans and urinary meatus (the opening for the passage of urine and semen).

When bacteria in the feces react with urine, they produce ammonia, which burns the skin and causes ammoniacal dermatitis, commonly known as diaper rash.

Other causes of a reddened foreskin are:

- too much exposure to soiled diapers
- an imbalance of skin bacteria caused by too many bubble baths or baby wipes
- overly chlorinated water (swimming pools, hot tubs)
- soap on the genitals
- laundry soap or detergent on clothing
- antibiotics (microbial flora can be restored by eating live culture yogurt)
- concentrated urine caused by not drinking enough water

The drinking of water, soaking in warm baths, and running around with a bare bottom help healing.

Remember that circumcision cannot prevent this redness. Without the superior protection of the foreskin, the diaper rash would appear on the delicate glans and meatus.

WHAT IS THE WHITE LUMP UNDER
MY SON'S FORESKIN?

The white lump is made up of the cells that once attached his foreskin to his glans. Some doctors mistakenly call these lumps "cysts." This is incorrect.

As new cells form on the glans and the foreskin's inside fold, old cells form "pockets" that eventually work their way to the tip of the foreskin, where they can simply be wiped away. The space they occupied becomes the preputial space between the foreskin and the glans. So, if you see a white lump under your son's foreskin, you know that the separation of his foreskin and glans is occurring naturally.

WHAT HAPPENS IF SOMEONE RETRACTS
MY SON'S FORESKIN PREMATURELY?

Forcing the foreskin back can be very painful and can cause problems. Tearing the foreskin from the glans leaves raw, open wounds, which can lead to infection. Raw surfaces on the foreskin and glans can heal together, forming adhesions. Small tears in the opening of the foreskin can heal to form nonelastic scar tissue, making it difficult to retract the foreskin later in life.

Doctors have made up some strange reasons for wanting to retract a child's foreskin during checkups. None of them are valid. They may sound convincing, but, I assure you, they are all wrong.

If a doctor tries to retract your child's foreskin, stop him. Tell him that this is inappropriate, unnecessary, and traumatic. Please, be on your guard. Many parents have made their feelings clear only to have doctors retract their son's foreskin anyway, causing the child enormous pain and trauma. Regardless of your child's age, and even if your child's foreskin is already fully retractable, doctors have no business fiddling with your child's penis and foreskin.

Sometimes they say they are looking for a urinary tract infection. This is absolutely ridiculous, but many doctors have actually said this to parents. Doctors who do this are usually circumcised and upset at the sight of an intact penis. They are unfamiliar with it and anxious. You know more than they do about this body part. You must take charge. Protect your child from any attempt to retract or tamper with his foreskin.

There are others besides ignorant doctors who ought to be instructed to leave the foreskin alone. It would be best to remind all baby-sitters and anyone else who cares for your child to avoid retracting his foreskin. Just a few days ago, a six-month-old baby boy was brought to my office with a swollen and extremely red foreskin with cuts covering all sides of his foreskin. The baby's parents had left their precious baby with a baby-sitter for the first time. She was unfamiliar with and confused by the sight of a normal human penis. While changing the baby's diapers, she became overzealous in cleaning his penis and imagined that she was supposed to retract his foreskin. Fortunately, his very sore penis will heal as long as it is left alone.

WHY DOES MY SON'S FORESKIN "BALLOON" WHEN HE URINATES?

This is another indication that the natural separation of his foreskin and glans is occurring. One European friend tells how as a boy, he and his friends, who were "lucky enough to have foreskins that ballooned," would stand in a row, urinate, then squeeze the balloon to see who could "shoot" the farthest. As the preputial opening widens, most boys decrease their chances of winning the game but increase their ability to retract their fore-skins.

Taking care of your child's intact penis is easy: Just leave your child's foreskin alone. It will take care of itself. Just as we never need to wash underneath our children's eyelids, so we never need to wash underneath the foreskin of a child. It is self-cleaning. Remember that your child's foreskin is supposed to be securely unretractable until he is a teenager. Finally, it is always best to protect your child from anyone who wants to retract his foreskin for any reason. Just tell your doctor to leave it alone.

Chapter Twelve

• ● •

Care of the Circumcised Penis

All of the western world raises its children uncircumcised and it seems logical that, with the extent of health knowledge in those countries, such a practice must be safe.[1]

C. Everett Koop, M.D.
former Surgeon General of the United States

There are going to be some parents who, for whatever reason, get talked into having their baby's penis circumcised. Many parents have asked me what method of circumcision would be best. It is my considered medical opinion, based on my experience as a pediatrician and based on my careful reading of the medical literature, that every method of circumcision presents its own unique set of risks and dangers. As we've seen in Chapter 3, the Plastibell method carries the highest risk of gangrene. The Gomco clamp can result in amputation of all of the skin of the penis. The Sheldon clamp is associated with accidental amputation of the glans as well as the foreskin. No method is safe, and every method results in a scarred, denuded, and desensitized penis. If you honestly feel that no amount of information or medical facts are sufficient to persuade you to protect your child from circumcision, the best advice I can offer is to seek out the services of the most highly qualified pediatric urological surgeon you can find. Also, I cannot stress enough the importance of insisting that the surgeon provide local anesthesia during and after the surgery. If the surgeon refuses or if he otherwise downplays or dismisses the importance of anesthesia, look for another surgeon. Circumcision is a serious operation. Your son's penis is at stake. If anything goes wrong, the consequences are likely to be tragic for your son and for your peace of mind.

Bearing this in mind, parents who contemplate subjecting their child to circumcision must be prepared to pay very close attention to the amputation wound. It will require careful watching and delicate handling lest infection or dangerous bleeding result.

Remember that before a baby's foreskin can be cut off, it must be forcibly *torn* from the glans with a metal probe. The entire glans of the baby's penis and the site of the incision are then raw, open wounds. If you have allowed a circumciser to talk you into letting him circumcise your baby, you must, therefore, watch your baby very carefully the first few days for possible complications.

Gomco Clamp Circumcision

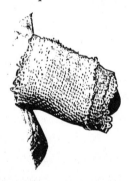

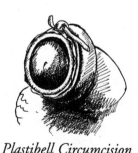

Plastibell Circumcision

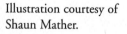
Illustration courtesy of
Shaun Mather.

WHAT POSTOPERATIVE COMPLICATIONS SHOULD I WATCH FOR?

Bleeding

After your baby is circumcised, bleeding is supposed to stop. Often, the bleeding continues, dangerously draining your baby of his life's blood. If your baby's penis keeps bleeding, the doctor should be notified immediately.

Infection

Infections can be in the wound, the tissue around the wound, the membrane just under the skin, and/or the bloodstream. Increasing redness, swelling, oozing, and fever are all signs of infection. Infections can quickly invade a newborn baby's body.

Infections can be deadly. If you see any sign of infection, the doctor should be notified immediately.

Urinary Retention

If your baby goes longer than eight hours without urinating after being circumcised, the doctor should be notified immediately.

Hypospadias and/or Urethral Fistula

If your baby's urinary opening (meatus) is somewhere other than the tip of the glans, or if urine comes out of any other opening in his penis, the doctor should be notified immediately.

Dislodged Plastibell Circumcision Device

If there is a plastic ring with a string tied around its rim on your baby's penis, it is supposed to drop off in five to eight days. If it fails to drop off within eight days, or if it slips from his glans onto his shaft, or if you notice any swelling, the doctor should be notified immediately.

Complications from Anesthetics

The penile dorsal nerve block requires injections into the base of the penis. Needles puncturing tissue in this area cause pain, and can cause bruising and can damage the dorsal penile nerve. Accidental puncture of the dorsal artery or vein can lead to hematoma or gangrene. If your baby has extensive bruising or swelling around the injection sites, the doctor should be notified.

Topical anesthetics, such as EMLA cream, fail to prevent circumcision pain. Furthermore, they carry the risk of methemoglobinemia (a type of blood poisoning in which hemoglobin cannot carry oxygen). If your baby's color turns bluish or grayish, or if he becomes lethargic, the doctor should be notified immediately.

Pain

After your baby is circumcised—with or without an anesthetic—he will be in excruciating pain. Urine and feces in the wound add to his discomfort and distress. Some doctors prescribe postoperative pain medication, but it is seldom effective and is never 100 percent effective.

It is very important to be cautious with the dose of pain medication, if any is given. Be sure to check that the dosage is correct by confirming it with your pediatrician, especially if the amputation was performed by a nonphysician circumciser. As for ritual Jewish circumcision, it is imperative that Jewish parents refrain from giving the baby more wine under the assumption that this will dull the pain. Personally, I cannot believe that sugar water provides analgesia, although I have heard it advocated by circumcisers who should know better.

Be sure to comfort your baby by holding him, nursing him frequently, sleeping with him, and being especially careful when changing his diapers. Babies who have recently been circumcised experience extreme pain and distress when their diapers are changed as a result of the disturbance to the surgical wound.[2]

WILL CIRCUMCISION CHANGE THE WAY MY BABY EATS OR SLEEPS?

Feeding

Some circumcised babies feed readily right after they are circumcised. Many are too shocked and traumatized to feed. These babies need more time to recover, usually several days.

Sleep Patterns

As you learned in Chapter 3, solid scientific research documents that circumcision disrupts normal sleep patterns. Having part of his penis cut off is a painful, stressful, and exhausting experience for a newborn baby. Many babies are unable to sleep properly after being circumcised. They spend more time awake, agitated, cranky, fussy, unable to feed, and in obvious pain. This may last for weeks. Hold your baby, comfort him, and nurse him whenever he wants.

HOW SHOULD I CARE FOR HIS CIRCUMCISION WOUND?

Dressing Changes

If your baby was circumcised with a Plastibell device, the plastic ring should be in place but there should be no dressing on his penis. The Plastibell device is supposed to fall off with the remnant foreskin once it has died, turned black, and separated from the body. This can take about a week. Please note that in many cases, the circumcision scar on a penis circumcised with a Plastibell will be dark and very noticeable. This additional disfigurement is permanent.

If your baby was circumcised with a Gomco clamp, his penis will be bandaged with a gauze dressing to keep the open wound on his remaining skin and the open wound on his glans from sticking to each other and to his diaper. Some doctors recommend replacing this dressing when it is soiled. Others recommend removing it after an hour or two. Some doctors recommend applying Vaseline to the wound with every diaper change to keep the wound from sticking to the diaper.

The yellowish crust on your baby's glans forms from the fluids that the body produces as part of the response to physical trauma and the healing process. It will fall off by itself as the glans heals.

Bathing

After your baby has a bowel movement, the circumcision area should be gently rinsed with warm running water. It is best to wait until the wound has healed (seven to ten days) before touching it or using a washcloth.

Preventing Adhesions

Adhesions form when new tissue grows between two structures that are normally separate. The raw surfaces of the glans and the remaining penile skin can fuse together. This can be prevented by pulling the penile shaft skin behind the line of incision gently away from the glans once or twice a day after the initial healing of the wound (seven to ten days). This should be done until your baby is at least one year old to ensure that the deeper layers of the wound heal without fusing to adjacent tissue.

If it should happen that adhesions form between the foreskin remnant and the raw glans, it is best simply to leave them alone. They will usually resolve themselves by the end of puberty.

WHAT ABOUT LATER COMPLICATIONS?

In Chapter 4, we examined many of the possible risks posed by circumcision. The following is a summary of the most frequent complications that are likely to develop during the first months and years of your child's life if you have him circumcised.

Meatitis

After circumcision, the urinary meatus no longer has its protective foreskin covering and may become irritated or infected, leading to meatitis (ulcers around the meatus). As the ulcers heal, scar tissue forms, constricting the meatus and causing a condition known as meatal stenosis.

Meatal Stenosis

Constriction of the meatus impedes and sometimes blocks the flow of urine. Urine backed up into the bladder can cause painful urination and obstructive renal disease. Urine retained in the bladder is a breeding ground for bacteria and can lead to infection. If you notice anything irregular about your baby's urine flow, the doctor should be notified. Surgery may be required to enlarge the urinary opening. (Meatal stenosis occurs almost exclusively among babies who have been circumcised.)

Preputial Stenosis

The circumcision scar sometimes forms as a tight, constricted, inelastic ring that traps the glans behind it. It may require corrective surgery.

Buried Penis

After circumcision, the penis may become entrapped by scar tissue and retract into the pubic fat and fascia. This condition may correct itself naturally but sometimes requires painful and disfiguring reconstructive surgery that leaves horrible scars on the abdomen and penis.

IS THERE ANYTHING ELSE I SHOULD KNOW?

Increasing numbers of males who were circumcised as babies are coming forward to report long-term circumcision-related complications. These include:

Discomfort

Some circumcised males find the constant abrasion of their exposed glans extremely uncomfortable.

Painful Erections

Males have erections throughout life, even before they are born. A male's foreskin provides exactly the right amount of skin necessary for his penis to experience comfortable erections. In a circumcision, so much penile skin is cut that some males experience painful erections. Unfortunately, it is impossible for the circumciser to determine whether he is cutting off too much skin. It all depends on how your son's penis develops and grows, and this cannot be predicted in infancy.

Scarring

Every circumcision results in a circular scar around the penis. Circumcision scars vary from male to male. Some are more noticeable than others. Many circumcised males feel self-conscious about the scar on their penis. Other circumcised males feel self-conscious that their glans is permanently externalized and has lost its normal coloration.

Desensitization

Anatomical research shows that the foreskin is erogenous tissue.[3] Cutting the foreskin off desensitizes the penis. Circumcision also causes the surface of the externalized glans to dry out, thicken, and toughen, causing even more desensitization. Many circumcised males have a hard time dealing with the realization that their penis has been permanently desensitized.

Chapter 13

●●●

Afterthoughts

Every medical society that has objectively examined the problem of circumcision has concluded that it is devoid of medical value. Unbiased scientists have settled the matter: circumcision is unnecessary, contraindicated, and harmful.

The foreskin has many useful and irreplaceable functions. Clearly, it is an important part of male anatomy that provides a lifetime of benefits to its owner. As an integral part of the penis from babyhood to the end of life, the foreskin keeps the penis clean, safe, healthy, warm, and sensitive. It allows the entire penis to complete its long development toward maturity in complete safety and without threat of interruption and premature cessation. The gliding motion of the foreskin up and down the shaft, the ability of the lips of the foreskin to open and close gently and easily, and the rich investment of nerves and blood vessels in the foreskin provide each male with a uniquely enhanced way of perceiving, experiencing, enjoying, and sharing his miraculous existence.

The fact that there are tens of thousands of sensory nerves in the normal foreskin explains why foreskin amputation is so excruciatingly painful and why modern medicine has repeatedly failed to develop a technique of local anesthesia that is completely safe and effective. The message should be very clear: Any procedure that causes that amount of extreme pain to an innocent newborn babe is clearly a mistake. A baby's agonizing and frenzied screams of pain are the only way he has to tell us to leave his penis alone and that he needs his foreskin to enjoy a life as a complete male. The principles of medical ethics require that we protect our babies from pain and trauma. If it is illegal to subject laboratory animals to painful experiences, what does it say about a society that would provide greater legal protection to lab rats than to its own children?

The principles of medical ethics require that we should protect and safeguard the foreskin and every male's right to sovereignty over it. It is a very serious matter to remove a functional part of the reproductive organ of the male. Even if the foreskin served no purpose, it would be improper to remove it from males without their permission. After all, whose penis is it? Sovereignty over one's own body is paramount.

Circumcisers—whether they be obstetricians, pediatricians, urologists, mohels, witch doctors, or barbers—are ignorant or in denial of *what* they are cutting off, even though they may be experts at *how* to cut it off. Surely, the principles of medical ethics are being violated by such ignorance, whether it be willful or not.

When we realize the very important functions of the intact penis, we are able to value the foreskin and appreciate nature's beautiful design for the human body. We will then have the intelligence to apply the wonders of modern medicine to find conservative and rational medical solutions to any medical problems that might arise in the life of the male, without resorting to primitive, antiquated, and outmoded surgical amputations. Modern medical techniques can now easily treat and solve any problem of the foreskin without surgery.

I am happy to report that the vast majority of parents want what is best for their baby. Parents want to do what is ethical and moral. Wise parents will listen to their hearts and trust their instinct to protect their baby from harm of any kind. The experience of the ages has shown that babies thrive best in a trusting atmosphere of love, gentleness, respect, acceptance, nurturing, and intimacy. Cutting off a baby's foreskin shatters this trust. Circumcision wounds and harms the baby and the person the baby will become. Parents who respect their son's wholeness are preserving for him his birthright—his intact body, perfect and beautiful in its entirety.

Children have the full rights of any human being. They are not partial humans. They are our ultimate investment. We must teach them compassion, peace, and trust if we want them, in the future, to be able to take care of us and our world with responsibility, reason, and loving kindness. History has shown that it is best to avoid inflicting any degree of pain, trauma, or violence on our children. Our society would be greatly improved and enhanced if circumcision, along with all other forms and degrees of injustice and violence against children, would stop. Studies consistently demonstrate that providing our infants and children with a home environment that is loving, safe, secure, compassionate, affectionate, nurturing, and orderly is the very best way to ensure that our children grow up to be reverent, moral, responsible, independent, self-confident, self-disciplined, secure, successful, rational, compassionate, and emotionally, physically, and mentally healthy adults of good character. Protecting our sons from circumcision and assuring that they enjoy the lifetime of natural benefits and protections that the intact human body can bring is part of the responsible parenting that produces responsible adults.

To paraphrase a pastoral letter from U.S. Catholic bishops,[1] every medical decision must be judged in light of whether it protects or undermines the dignity of the human person. Surgically removing the foreskin—or any other body part, for that matter—without absolute and urgent medical necessity from someone who has not been given the dignity of a choice in the matter necessarily undermines the human dignity of the violated person as well as those responsible for this violation. Every person and every part of every person is sacred. Human dignity comes from our human essence, not from nationality, race, religious affiliation, sex, economic status, or any human accomplishment. Human personhood must be respected with a reverence that is religious. When we deal with each other on any level—including medical—we should do so with the sense of awe that arises in the presence of something holy and sacred. The foreskin is a vital part of the perfection of the human body.

In closing, let me recall for you the fundamental truth that life is a blessing, and that every child and *every body part* of every child is sacred. Furthermore, as wise men of ancient times observed, the human body is a temple to the soul. Let us show the greatest reverence and respect for the bodily temple and rejoice in its every part and function by preserving it intact. Let us respect the wondrous discoveries of true science and respect human dignity. Our children are counting on us.

Appendix A:
Position Statements on Circumcision of National and International Medical Associations

The American Medical Association states:

The low incidence of urinary tract infections and penile cancer mitigates the potential medical benefits compared with the risks of circumcision. In the case of sexual transmission of HIV, behavioral factors are far more important in preventing these infections than the presence or absence of a foreskin.[1]

The American Academy of Pediatrics states:

Existing scientific evidence demonstrates potential medical benefits of newborn circumcision; however, these data are not sufficient to recommend routine neonatal circumcision.[2]

The American College of Obstetricians and Gynecologists states:

The American College of Obstetricians and Gynecologists supports the current position of the American Academy of Pediatrics that finds the existing evidence insufficient to recommend routine neonatal circumcision.[3]

The American Cancer Society states in a letter to the American Academy of Pediatrics:

We would like to discourage the American Academy of Pediatrics from promoting routine circumcision as a preventive measure for penile or cervical cancer. . . . Perpetuating the mistaken belief that circumcision prevents cancer is inappropriate.[4]

The Australasian Association of Paediatric Surgeons states:

It is considered to be inappropriate and unnecessary as a routine to remove the prepuce, based on the current evidence available.[5]

The Australian College of Paediatrics states:

Routine male circumcision should not be performed prior to 6 months of age. In addition, it considers that neonatal male circumcision has no medical indication. It is a traumatic procedure, performed without anaesthesia to remove a normal functional and protective prepuce.[6]

The British Medical Association Guidelines advise:

The BMA opposes unnecessarily invasive procedures being used where alternative, less invasive techniques, are equally efficient and available.[7]

The Canadian Paediatric Society recommends:

Circumcision of newborns should not be routinely performed.[8]

Appendix B:
Resources and Organizations

Organizations Serving the Needs of Parents

If your physician or health care provider ever recommends that your child be circumcised, get another opinion from a physician who understands the important functions of the foreskin, no matter how "urgent" the situation may be. For help finding one in your area and for a source of great information, contact:

National Organization of Circumcision Information Resource Centers (NOCIRC) International Headquarters. Marilyn Fayre Milos, RN, Executive Director, PO Box 2512, San Anselmo, CA 94979-2512 USA, tel: 415-488-9883, fax: 415-488-9660, www.nocirc.org

NOCIRC of Australia. George L. Williams, MD, POB 248, Menai 2234 NSW Australia, tel: 61-2-9543-0222. Also: Mervyn M. Lander, MD, 131 Wickham Terrace, Brisbane 4000, Queensland, Australia, tel: 7-3-839-4742, fax: 7-3-832-6674

Organizations Serving the Needs of Jewish Parents

Circumcision Resource Center. Ronald Goldman, Ph.D., PO Box 232, Boston, Massachusetts, 02133 USA, tel: 617-523-0088, www.circumcision.org

Organizations for Doctors

Doctors Opposing Circumcision (D.O.C.). George Denniston, MD, MPH, 2442 NW Market Street #42, Seattle, WA 98107 USA, tel: 360-385-1882, fax: 360-385-1965, http://weber.u.washington.edu/~gcd/DOC/

Organizations for Nurses

Nurses for the Rights of the Child. Mary Conant, RN, Betty Katz Sperlich, RN, Mary-Rose Booker, RN, 369 Montezuma #354, Santa Fe, New Mexico 87501 USA, tel: 505-989-7377, www.cirp.org/nrc

Organizations Serving the Needs of Circumcised Men

National Organization of Restoring Men (NORM) International Headquarters. R. Wayne Griffiths, MS, Med, 3505 Northwood Drive, Suite 209, Concord, CA 94520-4506 USA, tel: 510-827-4066, fax: 510-827-4119, www.norm.org

NORM-UK. John P. Warren, MB, Chairman, PO Box 71, Stone, Staffordshire, ST15 0SF, United Kingdom, tel/fax: 01785-814-044, www.norm-uk.co.uk

UnCircumcising Information and Resource Center (UN-CIRC). Jim Bigelow, Ph.D., PO Box 52138, Pacific Grove, CA 93950 USA, tel/fax: 408-375-4326

Organizations for Lawyers

Attorneys for the Rights of the Child. J. Steven Svoboda, JD. 2961 Ashby Ave, Berkeley, CA 94705 USA, fax/phone 510-595-5550. www.arclaw.org

Appendix C:
Recommended Reading

Web Sites for Parents

National Organization of Circumcision Information Resource
Centers (NOCIRC)
www.nocirc.org

The Circumcision Information and Resource Pages
www.cirp.org

Intact
www.intact.ca

Alliance for Transforming the Lives of Children
www.atlc.org

BoysToo.com (Official Web Site of NOCIRC of North
Dakota)
www.boystoo.com

Circumcision Information Resource Center (Montreal, Canada)
www.infocirc.org/index-e.htm

Circumcision Resource Center (Boston, Massachusetts)
www.circumcision.org

CIRCUMCISION: the virtual journal
http://weber.u.washington.edu/~gcd/CIRCUMCISION/

D.O.C. (Doctors Opposing Circumcision)
http://weber.u.washington.edu/~gcd/DOC/

In Memory of the Sexually Mutilated Child (John A. Erickson)
www.SexuallyMutilatedChild.org

International Coalition for Genital Integrity
www.icgi.org

Mothers Against Circumcision
http://members.aol.com/maggimagoo/index.html

National Organization to Halt the Abuse and Routine Mutilation of Males (NOHARMM)
www.noharmm.org

City of Light
www.moslem.org

Web Sites on Foreskin Restoration

National Organization of Restoring Men (NORM)
www.norm.org

NORM-UK (Great Britain)
www.norm-uk.co.uk

Web Sites for Lawyers

Attorneys for the Rights of the Child
www.arclaw.org

Books for Parents

Billy Ray Boyd. *Circumcision Exposed: Rethinking a Medical and Cultural Tradition.* Freedom, CA: The Crossing Press, 1998. [IBSN 0-89594-939-3]

Anne Briggs. *Circumcision: What Every Parent Should Know.* Charlottesville, VA: Birth & Parenting Publications, 1985. [ISBN 0-9615484-0-1]

John Colapinto. *As Nature Made Him: The Boy Who Was Raised as a Girl.* New York: HarperCollins, 2000. [ISBN 0-06-019211-9]

Ronald Goldman, Ph.D. *Circumcision: The Hidden Trauma.* Boston: Vanguard, 1996. [IBSN 0-9644895-3-8]

Peggy O'Mara, ed. *Circumcision: The Rest of the Story.* Santa Fe, NM: Mothering, 1993. [ISBN 0-914257-11-0]

Thomas J. Ritter, MD, and George C. Denniston, MD. *Doctors Re-examine Circumcision.* Aptos, CA: Third Millenium Publishing Company, 2001. [ISBN 0-971187800]

Rosemary Romberg. *Circumcision: The Painful Dilemma.* South Hadley, MA: Bergan & Garvey, 1985. [ISBN 0897890736]

Edward Wallerstein. *Circumcision: An American Health Fallacy.* New York. Springer, 1980. [ISBN 0826132405]

Books for Jewish Parents

Ronald Goldman, Ph.D. *Questioning Circumcision: A Jewish Perspective.* Boston: Vanguard, 1997. [ISBN 0-9644895-6-2]

Kayla Weiner, Ph.D., and Arinna Moon, MA., eds. *Jewish Women Speak Out: Expanding the Boundaries of Psychology.* Seattle, WA: Canopy Press, 1995. [ISBN 0964587807]

Books on Foreskin Restoration

Jim Bigelow, PhD. *The Joy of Uncircumcising!* 2nd edition. Aptos, CA: Hourglass, 1995. [ISBN 0-934061-22-x]

Books for Doctors, Scholars, and Those Who Want More Information

George C. Denniston and Marilyn Fayre Milos, eds. *Sexual Mutilations: A Human Tragedy.* New York and London: Plenum Publishing Corporation, 1997. [ISBN 0-3-6-45589-7]

George C. Denniston, Frederick Mansfield Hodges and Marilyn Fayre Milos, eds. *Male and Female Circumcision: Medical, Legal, and Ethical Considerations in Pediatric Practice.* New York, Boston, Dordrecht, London, Moscow: Kluwer Academic/Plenum Publishers, 1999. [ISBN 0-306-46131-5]

George C. Denniston, Frederick Mansfield Hodges and Marilyn Fayre Milos, eds. *Understanding Circumcision: A Multi-Disciplinary Approach to a Multi-Dimensional Problem.* New York: Kluwer Academic/Plenum Publishers, 2001. [ISBN 0-306-46701-1]

David L. Gollaher. *Circumcision: A History of the World's Most Controversial Surgery.* New York: Basic Books, 2000. [ISBN 0-456-04397-6]

Kristen O'Hara with Jeffrey O'Hara. *Sex As Nature Intended It.* Hudson, MA: Turning Point Publications, 2001. [ISBN 0-9700442-0-8]

Margaret Somerville. *The Ethical Canary: Science, Society and the Human Spirit.* Toronto: Penguin, 2000. [ISBN 0-670-89971-2]

Sami A. Aldeeb Abu-Sahlieh. *Male Circumcision and Female Circumcision Among Jews, Christians and Muslims: Religious,*

Medical, Social and Legal Debate. Marco Polo Monographs 5. Warren Centre, Pennsylvania: Shangri-La Publications, 2001. [ISBN 0-9677201-8-2]

Videotapes/Films

Facing Circumcision: Eight Physicians Tell Their Stories and Reveal the Ethical Dilemmas of Physicians Who Circumcise Newborns. Nurses for the Rights of the Child. 20 minutes. VHS. 1998. Nurses for the Rights of the Child. 369 Montezuma #354, Santa Fe, New Mexico, 87501, 505-989-7377, *www.cirp.org/nrc*

It's a Boy! Victor Schonfeld. 41 minutes. VHS. $295 institutions, $195 individuals, $65 rental. Filmmakers Library, 124 East 40th Street, New York, NY 10016, tel: 212-808-4980, fax: 212-808-4983.

The Nurses of St. Vincent: Saying "No" to Circumcision. Barry Ellsworth. Includes NOHARMM Rally at California Medical Association. VHS. 30 minutes. $29. NOCIRC, POB 2512, San Anselmo, CA 94979.

Prince for a Day: The Sumbawa Circumcision Ceremony. Royal Phillips. VHS. $30. Book $10. Royal Productions, POB 40150, Santa Barbara, CA 93103.

Whose Body, Whose Rights? Lawrence Dillon and Tim Hammond. 1996. 56 minutes. VHS. Home Sales: Video-Finders, 1-800-343-4727. Educational Sales: $195, Rental $70, Catalogue #38342, University of California Extension,

Center for Media and Independent Learning, 2000 Center Street, Fourth Floor, Berkeley, CA 94704, 510-642-0460.

Newsletters

NOCIRC Annual Report. Marilyn Fayre Milos, RN, editor, NOCIRC. POB 2512. San Anselmo, CA 94979-2512, USA

NOCIRC of Michigan Informant. Norm Cohen, editor, POB 333, Birmingham, MI 48012

NOCIRC Newsletter of Australia. Dr. George Williams, editor, NOCIRC of Australia, POB 248, Menai Central, NSW 2234 Australia.

Source Notes

Introduction

1. Adler R, Ottaway S, Gould S. Circumcision: we have heard from the experts; now let's hear from the parents. Pediatrics 2001 Feb;107(2):E20.

2. Shaw RA, Robertson WO. Routine circumcision: A problem for medicine. Am J DB Child 1963 Aug;106(2):216–7.

3. HCIA-Sachs. Circumcision of American babies declines 11 percent in just five years. HCIA.com (Thursday, 13 May 1999). URL: http://www.hcia.com/findings/990513_circum.htm#1993

Chapter 1: What Is the Foreskin?

1. Cold CJ, Taylor JR. The prepuce. BJU Int 1999 Jan; 83:34–44. [here, p. 34].

2. Hodges FM. The ideal prepuce in ancient Greece and Rome: male genital aesthetics and their relation to lipodermos, circumcision, foreskin restoration, and the kynodesmé. Bull Hist Med 2001;75:375–405.

3. See photographic series in: Lander MM. The human prepuce. In: Denniston GC, Milos MF (eds). Sexual Mutilations: A Human Tragedy. New York: Plenum Press; 1997. pp. 79–81.

See Photograph 1 in: Davenport M. Problems with the penis and prepuce: natural history of the foreskin. BMJ 1996;312:299–301.

4. Jefferson G. The peripenic muscle; some observations on the anatomy of phimosis. Surgery, Gynecology and Obstetrics 1916 Aug;23(2):177–81.

5. Parkash S, Jeyakumar S, Subramanyan K, Chaudhuri S. Human subpreputial collection: its nature and formation. J Urol 1973 Aug; 110(2): 211–2.

Lakshmanan S, Parkash S. Human prepuce: some aspects of structure and function. Ind J Surg 1980 Mar;42(3):134–7.

6. Hyman AB, Brownstein MH. Tyson's "glands": ectopic sebaceous glands and papillomatosis penis. Arch Dermatol 1969 Jan;99(1):31–6.

Ahmed A, Jones AW. Apocrine cystadenoma. A report of two cases occurring on the prepuce. Br J Dermatol 1969 Dec;81(12):899–901.

7. Taylor JR, Lockwood AP, Taylor AJ. The prepuce: specialized mucosa of the penis and its loss to circumcision. Br J Urol 1996 Feb;77(2): 291–5.

8. Diebert GA. The separation of the prepuce in the human penis. Anatomical Record 1933 Nov;57(4):387–99.

Hunter RH. Notes on the development of the prepuce. Journal of Anatomy 1935 Oct;70(1):68–75.

Gairdner D. The fate of the foreskin. BMJ 1949 Dec 24;2(4642): 1433–7.

Glenister TW. A consideration of the processes involved in the development of the prepuce in man. Br J Urol 1956 Sep;28(3):243–9.

9. Oster J. Further fate of the foreskin. Incidence of preputial adhesions, phimosis, and smegma among Danish schoolboys. Arch Dis Child 1968 Apr;43(228):200–3.

Kayaba H, Tamura H, Kitajima S, Fujiwara Y, Kato T. Analysis of shape and rectractability of the prepuce in 603 Japanese boys. J Urol 1996 Nov;156(5):1813–5.

10. Salesses A, Rabineau D. [Histologic study of the individualization of the prepuce in man]. Arch Anat Pathol (Paris) 1965 June;13(2):114–8.

11. Parkash S, Rao R, Venkatesan K, Ramafrishnan S. Sub-preputial wetness: its nature. Ann Natl Med Sci (India) 1982 Jul–Sep;18(3):109–12.

12. Koning M, Streekferk J.G. Kleine kwalen in de huisartsgeneeskunde; smegma en fysiologische fimose, Nederlands Tijdschrift voor Geeneskunde, 1995 Aug 12;139(32):1632–4.

13. Parkash S, Jeyakumar S, Subramanyan K, Chaudhuri S. Human subpreputial collection: its nature and formation. J Urol 1973 Aug;110(2): 211–2.

Parkash S, Rao R, Venkatesan K, Ramakirshnan S. Sub-preputial wetness: its nature. Ann Natl Med Sci 1982 Jul–Sep;18(3):109–12.

14. Ritter TJ, Denniston GC. Say No to Circumcision: 40 Compelling Reasons. 2nd ed. Aptos, CA: Hourglass; 1996. p. 6:2.

15. Coppa GV, Gabrielli O, Giorgi P, Catassi C, Montanari MP, Varaldo PE, Nichols BL. Preliminary study of breastfeeding and bacterial adhesion to uroepithelial cells. Lancet 1990 Mar 10;335(8689):569–71.

16. Flower PJ, Ladds PW, Thomas AD, Watson DL. An immunopathologic study of the bovine prepuce. Vet Pathol 1983 Mar; 20(2):189–202.

17. Moldwin RM, Valderrama E. Immunohistochemical analysis of nerve distribution patterns within preputial tissues. J Urol 1989 Apr;141(4):499A. (Abstract)

18. Taylor JR, Lockwood AP, Taylor AJ. The prepuce: specialized mucosa of the penis and its loss to circumcision. Br J Urol 1996 Feb;77(2):291–5.

19. Dogiel AS. Die Nervenendigungen in der Haut der äusseren Genitalorgane des Menschen. Archiv für Mikroskopische Anatomie 1893:41:585–612.

Bazett HC, McGlone B, Williams RG, Lufkin HM. Depth, distribution and probable identification in the prepuce of sensory end-organs concerned in sensations of temperature and touch; thermometric conductivity. Archives of Neurology and Psychiatry 1932 Mar;27(3):489–517.

20. Bazett HC, McGlone B, Williams RG, Lufkin HM. Depth, distribution and probable identification in the prepuce of sensory end-organs concerned in sensations of temperature and touch; thermometric conductivity. Archives of Neurology and Psychiatry 1932 Mar;27(3):489–517.

21. Ohmori D. Über die Entwicklung der Innervation der Genitalapparate als peripheren Aufnahmeapparat der Genitalen Reflexe. Zeitschrift für Anatomie und Entwicklungsgeschichte 1924;70(1):347–410.

22. Halata Z, Munger BL. The neuroanatomical basis for the protopathic sensibility of the human glans penis. Brain Res 1986 Apr 23;371(2):205–30.

23. Ohmori D. Über die Entwicklung der Innervation der Genitalapparate als peripheren Aufnahmeapparat der Genitalen Reflexe. Zeitschrift für Anatomie und Entwicklungsgeschichte 1924:70(1):347–410.

24. Ohmori D. Über die Entwicklung der Innervation der Genitalapparate als peripheren Aufnahmeapparat der Genitalen Reflexe. Zeitschrift für Anatomie und Entwicklungsgeschichte 1924:70(1):347–410.

25. Winkelmann RK. The cutaneous innervation of human newborn prepuce. Invest Dermatol 1956 Jan;26(1):53–67.

26. Winkelmann RK. The erogenous zones: their nerve supply and its significance. Proceedings of the Staff Meetings of the Mayo Clinic 1959 Jan 21:34(2):39–47.

27. Halata Z, Munger BL. The neuroanatomical basis for the proto-pathic sensibility of the human glans penis. Brain Res 1986 Apr 23;371(2):205–30.

28. Taylor JR, Lockwood AP, Taylor AJ. The prepuce: specialized mu-cosa of the penis and its loss to circumcision. Br J Urol 1996 Feb;77(2): 291–5.

29. Cold CJ, McGrath KA. Anatomy and histology of the penile and clitoral prepuce in primates: an evolutionary perspective of the specialized sensory tissue of the external genitalia. In: Denniston GC, Hodges MF, Milos FM (eds). Male and Female Circumcision: Medical, Legal, and Ethi-cal Considerations in Pediatric Practice. New York: Kluwer Academic/ Plenum Publishers, 1999. pp. 19–29.

Chapter 2: The Functions of the Foreskin

1. Cold CJ, Taylor JR. The prepuce. BJU Int 1999 Jan; 83:34–44 [here, p. 41].

2. Hyman AB, Brownstein MH. Tyson's "glands": ectopic sebaceous glands and papillomatosis penis. Arch Dermatol 1969 Jan;99(1):31–6.

3. Parkash S, Jeyakumar S, Subramanyan K, Chaudhuri S. Human sub-preputial collection: its nature and formation. J Urol 1973 Aug; 110(2):211–2.

4. Parkash S. Penis: some facts and fancies. Journal of Physician's Asso-ciation of Madras June 1982: pp. 1–13.

5. Ahmed A, Jones AW. Apocrine cystadenoma: a report of two cases oc-curring on the prepuce. Br J Dermatol 1969 Dec;81(12):899–901.

6. Weiss GN, Sanders M, Westbrook KC. The distribution and density of Langerhans cells in the human prepuce: site of a diminished immune re-sponse? Isr J Med Sci 1993 Jan;29(1):42–3.

7. Flower PJ, Ladds PW, Thomas AD, Watson DL. An immunopatho-logic study of the bovine prepuce. Vet Pathol 1983 Mar;20(2):189–202.

8. Cook LS, Koutsky LA, Holmes KK. Clinical presentation of genital

warts among circumcised and uncircumcised heterosexual men attending an urban STD clinic. Genitourin Med 1993 Aug;69(4):262–4.

Smith GL, Greenup R, Takafuji ET. Circumcision as a risk factor for urethritis in racial groups. Am J Public Health 1987 Apr;77(4):452–4.

Aynaud O, Ionesco M, Barrasso R. Penile intraepithelial neoplasia: specific clinical features correlate with histologic and virologic findings. Cancer 1994 Sep 15;74(6):1762–7.

Donovan B, Bassett I, Bodsworth NJ. Male circumcision and common sexually transmissible diseases in a developed nation setting. Genitourin Med 1994 Oct;70(5):317–20.

Bassett I, Donovan B, Bodsworth NJ, Field PR, Ho DW, Jeansson S, Cunningham AL. Herpes simplex virus type 2 infection of heterosexual men attending a sexual health centre. Med J Aust 1994 Jun 6;160(11):697–700.

9. Hanson LA, Karlsson B, Jalil F, et al. Antiviral and antibacterial factors in human milk. In: Hanson LA, ed. Biology of Human Milk. New York: Raven Press; 1988. pp. 141–57.

May JT. Microbial contaminants and antimicrobial properties of human milk. Microbiol Sci 1988 Feb;5(2):42–6.

10. Coppa GV, Gabrielli O, Giorgi P, Catassi C, Montanari MP, Varaldo PE, Nichols BL. Preliminary study of breastfeeding and bacterial adhesion to uroepithelial cells. Lancet 1990 Mar 10;335(8689):569–71.

11. Flower PJ, Ladds PW, Thomas AD, Watson DL. An immunopathologic study of the bovine prepuce. Vet Pathol 1983 Mar;20(2):189–202.

12. Ahmed A, Jones AW. Apocrine cystadenoma: a report of two cases occurring on the prepuce. Br J Dermatol 1969 Dec;81(12):899–901.

13. Frohlich E, Schaumburg-Lever G, Klessen C. Immunelectron microscopic localization of cathepsin B in human exocrine glands. J Cutan Pathol 1993 Feb;20(1):54–60.

14. Ahmed AA, Nordlind K, Schultzberg M, Liden S. Immunohistochemical localization of IL-1 alpha-, IL-1 beta-, IL-6- and TNF-alpha-like immunoreactivities in human apocrine glands. Arch Dermatol Res 1995;287(8):764–6.

15. Halata Z, Munger BL. The neuroanatomical basis for the protopathic sensibility of the human glans penis. Brain Res 1986 Apr 23;371(2):205–30.

16. Taylor JR, Lockwood AP, Taylor AJ. The prepuce: specialized mucosa of the penis and its loss to circumcision. Br J Urol 1996 Feb;77(2):291–5.

Bazett HC, McGlone B, Williams RG, Lufkin HM. Depth, distribution and probable identification in the prepuce of sensory end-organs concerned in sensations of temperature and touch; thermometric conductivity. Arch Neurol and Psych 1932 Mar;27(3):489–517.

Ohmori D. Über die Entwicklung der Innervation der Genitalapparate als peripheren Aufnahmeapparat der Genitalen Reflexe. Zeitschrift für Anatomie und Entwicklungsgeschichte 1924;70(1):347–410.

De Girolamo A, Cecio A. [Contribution to the knowledge of sensory innervation of the prepuce in man]. Boll Soc Ital Biol Sper 1968 Sep 30;44(18):1521–2.

Dogiel AS. Die Nervenendigungen in der Haut der äusseren Genitalorgane des Menschen. Archiv für Mikroskopische Anatomie 1893; 41: 585–612.

Bourlond A, Winkelmann RK. [The innervation of the prepuce of the newborn infant]. Arch Belg Dermatol Syphiligr 1965 Oct;21(2):139–53.

Winkelmann RK. The cutaneous innervation of human newborn prepuce. Invest Dermatol 1956 Jan;26(1):53–67.

Winkelmann RK. The erogenous zones: their nerve supply and its significance. Proceedings of the Staff Meetings of the Mayo Clinic 1959 Jan 21;34(2):39–47.

17. Cohn BA. In search of human skin pheromones. Arch Dermatol 1994 Aug;130(8):1048–51.

18. Berliner DL, Jennings-White C, Lavker RM. The human skin: fragrances and pheromones. J Steroid Biochem Mol Biol 1991 Oct;39(4B): 671–9.

Chapter 3: What Happens to a Baby During a Circumcision?

1. Otten C. The case against newborn circumcision. Saturday Evening Post 1981 Dec;253(9):30–1, 116.

2. Cited in: Goldman R. The psychological impact of circumcision. BJU Int 1999 Jan;83 Suppl 1:93–102 [here, p. 94].

3. Cited in: Goldman R. The psychological impact of circumcision. BJU Int 1999 Jan;83 Suppl 1:93–102 [here, p. 94].

4. Grimes DA. Routine circumcision of the newborn infant: a reappraisal. Am J Obstet Gynecol 1978 Jan 15;130(2):125–9.

5. Holman JR, Lewis EL, Ringler RL. Neonatal circumcision techniques. American Family Physician 1995 Aug;52(2):511–8.

6. Porter FL, Porges SW, Marshall RW. Newborn pain cries and vagal tone: parallel changes in response to circumcision. Child Development 1988 Apr;59(2):495–505.

7. Yellen HS. Bloodless circumcision of the newborn. Am J Obstet Gynecol 1935 Jul;30(1):146–7.

8. Gunnar MR, Fisch RO, Korsvik S, Donhowe JM. The effects of circumcision on serum cortisol and behavior. Psychoneuroendocrinology 1981; 6(3)269–75.

9. Gee WF, Ansell JS. Neonatal circumcision: a ten-year overview: with comparison of the Gomco clamp and the Plastibell device. Pediatrics 1976 Dec;58(6):824–7.

Kaplan GW. Complications of circumcision. Urol Clin North Am 1983 Aug;10(3):543–9.

10. ECRI Problem Reporting System. Damaged Allied Healthcare Products, Gomco circumcision clamps. Health Devices 1993 Mar;22(3): 154–5.

11. Rubenstein MM, Bason WM. Complication of circumcision done with a plastic bell clamp. Am J Dis Child 1968 Oct;116(4):381–2.

Malo T, Bonforte RJ. Hazards of plastic bell circumcision. Obstet Gynecol 1969 Jun;33(6):869.

Datta NS, Zinner NR. Complication from Plastibell circumcision ring. Urology 1977 Jan;9(1):57–8.

Johnsonbaugh RE, Meyer BP, Catalano JD. Complication of a circumcision performed with a plastic bell clamp. Am J Dis Child 1969 Nov;118(5):781.

Jonas G. Retention of a Plastibell circumcision ring: report of a case. Obstet Gynecol 1984 Dec;24(6):835.

Stranko J, Ryan ME, Bowman Am. Impetigo in newborn infants associated with a plastic bell clamp circumcision. Pediatr Infect Dis 1986 Sep–Oct;5(5):597–9.

Sorensen SM, Sorensen MR. Circumcision with the Plastibell device: a long-term followup. Int Urol Nephrol 1988;20(2):159–66.

Wiswell TE, Curtis J, Dobek AS, Zierdt CH. Staphylococcus aureus colonization after neonatal circumcision in relation to device used. J Pediatr 1991 Aug;119(2):302–4.

Lee LD, Millar AJW. Ruptured bladder following circumcision using the Plastibell device. Br J Urol 1990 Feb;65(2):216–7.

12. Johnsonbaugh RE, Meyer BP, Catalano JD. Complication of a circumcision performed with a plastic bell clamp. Am J Dis Child 1969 Nov;118(5):781.

13. Orozco-Sanchez J, Neri-Vela R. [Total denudation of the penis in circumcision: description of a plastic technique for repair of the penis]. Bol Med Hosp Infant Mex 1991 Aug;48(8):565–9.

14. Datta NS, Zinner NR. Complication from Plastibell circumcision ring. Urology 1977 Jan;9(1):57–8.

Mihssin N, Moorthy K, Houghton PW. Retention of urine: an unusual complication of the Plastibell device. BJU Int 1999 Oct;84(6):745.

Rosefsky JB. Glans necrosis as a complication of circumcision. Pediatrics 1967 May;39(5):774–6.

Bliss DP, Healey PJ, Waldhausen JHT. Necrotizing fasciitis after Plastibell circumcision. J Pediatr 1997 Sep;31(3):459–62.

15. Gee WF, Ansell JS. Neonatal circumcision: a ten-year overview: with comparison of the Gomco clamp and the Plastibell device. Pediatrics 1976 Dec;58(6):824–7.

16. Woodside JR. Necrotizing fasciitis after neonatal circumcision. Am J Dis Child 1980 Mar;134(3):301–2.

17. Pearlman CK. Reconstruction following iatrogenic burn of the penis. J Pediatr Surg 1976 Feb;11(1):121–2.

18. Gearhart JP, Rock JA. Total ablation of the penis after circumcision with electrocautery: a method of management and long-term followup. J Urol 1989 Sep;142(3):799–801.

19. John Colapinto. As Nature Made Him: The Boy Who Was Raised as a Girl. New York: HarperCollins. 2000.

20. Strimling BS. Partial amputation of glans penis during Mogen clamp circumcision. Pediatrics 1996 June;97(6 Pt 1):906–7.

Sherman J, Borer JG, Horowitz M, Glassberg KI. Circumcision: successful glanular reconstruction and survival following traumatic amputation. J Urol 1996 Aug;156(2 Pt 2):842–4.

21. Gluckman GR, Stoller ML, Jacobs MM, Kogan BA. Newborn penile glans amputation during circumcision and successful reattachment. J Urol 1995 Mar;153(3 Pt 1):778–9.

22. Lander J, Brady-Fryer B, Metcalfe, JB, Nazarali S, Muttitt S. Comparison of ring block, dorsal penile nerve block, and topical anesthesia for

neonatal circumcision: a randomized controlled trial. JAMA 1997 Dec 24–31;278(24):2157–62.

23. Sara CA, Lowry CJ. A complication of circumcision and dorsal nerve block of the penis. Anaesth Intensive Care 1985 Feb;13(1):79–82.

24. Berens R, Pontus SP Jr. A complication associated with dorsal penile nerve block. Reg Anesth 1990 Nov–Dec;15(6):309–10.

25. Snellman LW, Stang HJ. Prospective evaluation of complications of dorsal penile nerve block for neonatal circumcision. Pediatrics 1995 May;95(5):705–8.

26. Van Howe RS. Anaesthesia for circumcision: a review of the literature. In: Denniston GC, Hodges FM, Milos MF (eds). Male and Female Circumcision: Medical, Legal, and Ethical Considerations in Pediatric Practice. New York: Kluwer Academic/Plenum Publishers, 1999. pp. 67–97.

27. Anand KJ, Hickey PR. Pain and its effects in the human neonate and fetus. N Engl J Med 1987 Nov 19;317(21):1321–9.

28. Taddio A, Goldbach M, Ipp M, Stevens B, Koren G. Effect of neonatal circumcision on pain responses during vaccination in boys. Lancet 1995 Feb 4;345(8945):291–2.

Taddio A, Katz J, Ilersich AL, Koren G. Effect of neonatal circumcision on pain response during subsequent routine vaccination. Lancet 1997 Mar 1:349(9052):599–603.

Taddio A, Stevens B, Craig K, Rastogi P, Ben-David S, Shennan A, Mulligan P, Koren G. Efficacy and safety of lidocaine-prilocaine cream for pain during circumcision. N Engl J Med 1997 Apr 24:336(17):1197–201.

Taddio A, Ohlsson A, Einarson TR, Stevens B, Koren G. A systematic review of lidocaine-prilocaine cream (EMLA) in the treatment of acute pain in neonates. Pediatrics 1998 Feb;101(2):E1.

Taddio A, Ohlsson K, Ohlsson A. Lidocaine-prilocaine cream for analgesia during circumcision in newborn boys. Cochrane Database Syst Rev 2000;(2):CD000496.

Taddio A, Pollock N, Gilbert-MacLeod C, Ohlsson K, Koren G. Combined analgesia and local anesthesia to minimize pain during circumcision. Arch Pediatr Adolesc Med 2000 Jun;154(6):620–3.

Taddio A. Pain management for neonatal circumcision. Paediatr Drugs 2001;3(2):101–11.

29. Prescott JW. Genital pain vs. genital pleasure: why the one and not the other? Truth Seeker 1989 Jul–Aug;1(3):14–21.

Prescott JW. Body pleasure and the origins of violence. Bull Atom Sci 1975 Nov;31(9):10–20.

30. Prescott JW. Genital pain vs. genital pleasure: why the one and not the other? Truth Seeker 1989 Jul–Aug;1(3):14–21.

31. Howard CR, Howard FM, Weitzman ML. Acetaminophen analgesia in neonatal circumcision: the effect on pain. Pediatrics 1994 Apr;93(4): 641–6.

32. Circumcision policy statement. American Academy of Pediatrics. Task Force on Circumcision. Pediatrics 1999 Mar;103(3):686–93.

33. Garry T. Circumcision: a survey of fees and practices. OBG Management 1994 Oct;6(10):34–6.

Stang HJ, Snellman LW. Circumcision practice patterns in the United States. Pediatrics 1998 Jun;101(6):E5.

Howard CR, Howard FM, Garfunkel LC, de Blieck EA, Weitzman M. Neonatal circumcision and pain relief: current training practices. Pediatrics 1998 Mar;101(3 Pt 1):423–8.

34. Stern E, Parmelee AH, Akiyama Y, Schultz MA, Wenner WH. Sleep cycle characteristics in infants. Pediatrics 1969 Jan;43(1):65–70.

35. Gunnar MR, Fisch RO, Korsvik S, Donhowe JM. The effects of circumcision on serum cortisol and behavior. Psychoneuroendocrinology 1981;6(3):269–75.

Gunnar MR, Fisch RO, Malone S. The effects of a pacifying stimulus on behavioral and adrenocortical responses to circumcision in the newborn. J Am Acad Child Psych 1984 Jan;23(1):34–8.

36. Anders TF, Chalemian RJ. The effects of circumcision on sleep-wake states in human neonates. Psychosom Med 1974 Mar–Apr;36(2):174–9.

37. Emde RN, Harmon RJ, Metcalf D, Koenig KL, Wagonfeld S. Stress and neonatal sleep. Psychosom Med 1971 Nov–Dec;33(6):491–7.

38. Marshall RE, Porter FL, Rogers AG, Moore J, Anderson B, Boxerman SB. Circumcision: II. Effects upon mother-infant interaction. Early Hum Dev 1982 Dec;7(4):367–74.

Dixon S, Snyder J, Holve R, Bromberger P. Behavioral effects of circumcision with and without anesthesia. J Dev Behav Pediatr 1984 Oct;5(5):246–50.

39. Marshall RE, Porter FL, Rogers AG, Moore J, Anderson B, Boxerman SB. Circumcision: II. Effects upon mother-infant interaction. Early Hum Dev 1982 Dec;7(4):367–74.

40. Dixon S, Snyder J, Holve R, Bromberger P. Behavioral effects of cir-

cumcision with and without anesthesia. J Dev Behav Pediatr 1984 Oct:5(5):246–50.

41. Howard CR, Howard FM, Weitzman ML. Acetaminophen analgesia in neonatal circumcision: the effect on pain. Pediatrics 1994 Apr;93(4): 641–6.

42. Dixon S, Snyder J, Holve R, Bromberger P. Behavioral effects of circumcision with and without anesthesia. J Dev Behav Pediatr 1984 Oct;5(5):246–50.

43. Marshall RE, Porter FL, Rogers AG, Moore J, Anderson B, Boxerman SB. Circumcision: II. Effects upon mother-infant interaction. Early Hum Dev 1982 Dec;7(4): 367–74.

44. Weissbluth M, Davis AT, Poncher J. Night waking in 4- to 8-month-old infants. J Pediatr 1984 Mar;104(3):477–80.

45. Anders TF. Night-waking in infants during the first year of life. Pediatrics 1979 Jun;63(6):860–4.

Chapter 4: Proven Complications and Risks of Circumcision

1. Snyder JL. The problem of circumcision in America. Truth Seeker 1989 Jul–Aug;1(3):39–42.

2. Williams N, Kapila L. Complications of circumcision. Br J Surg 1993 Oct;1993;80:1231–6.

3. Gee WF. Ansell JS. Neonatal circumcision: a ten-year overview: with comparison of the Gomco clamp and the Plastibell device. Pediatrics 1976 Dec;58(6):824–7.

4. Fletcher C. cited in: Fauntleroy G. Infant circumcision: the debate over parents' rights, human rights and the right to choose. Santa Fe New Mexican (30 July 2001): URL: http://www.sfnewmexican.com

5. Metcalf TJ, Osborn LM, Mariani EM. Circumcision: a study of current practices. Clin Pediatr (Phila) 1983 Aug;22(8):575–9.

Leitch IOW. Circumcision: a continuing enigma. Aust Paediatr J 1970 Mar;6(2):59–65.

Griffiths DM. Atwell JD. Freeman NV. A prospective survey of the indications and morbidity of circumcision in children. Eur Urol 1985;11(3): 184–7.

Fergusson DM, Lawton JM, Shannon FT. Neonatal circumcision and penile problems: an 8-year longitudinal study. Pediatrics 1988 Apr;81(4): 537–41.

Ozdemir E. Significantly increased complication risk with mass circumcisions. Br J Urol 1997 Jul;80(6):136–9.

6. Patel H. The problem of routine circumcision. Can Med Assoc J 1996 Sep 10;95(11):576–81.

7. Fraser IA, Allen MJ, Bagshaw PF, Johnstone M. A randomized trial to assess childhood circumcision with the Plastibell device compared to a conventional dissection technique. Br J Surg 1981 Aug;68(8):593–5.

Fredman RM. Neonatal circumcision: a general practitioner survey. Med J Aust 1969 Jan 18:1(3):117–20.

Gee WF, Ansell JS. Neonatal circumcision: a ten-year overview: with comparison of the Gomco clamp and the Plastibell device. Pediatrics 1976 Dec;58(6):824–7.

Hovsepian D. The pros and cons of routine circumcision. Calif Med 1951 Nov;75(5):359–61.

Patel H. The problem of routine circumcision. Can Med Assoc J 1966 Sep 10;95(11):576–81.

Shulman J, Ben-Hur N, Neuman Z. Surgical complications of circumcision. Am J Dis Child 1964 Feb;107(2):149–54.

8. Van Duyn J. quoted in: Circumcision is still given loud yeas and nays: advocates say procedure lowers incidence of cancer; opponents call the population statistics misleading. Medical Tribune 1965 Jun 12–13;6(70):7.

9. Fraser IA, Allen MJ, Bagshaw PF, Johnstone M. A randomized trial to assess childhood circumcision with the Plastibell device compared to a conventional dissection technique. Br J. Surg 1981 Aug;68(8):593–5.

Williams N, Kapila L. Complications of circumcision. Br J Surg 1993 Oct;1993;80:1231–6.

10. Gosden M. Tetanus following circumcision. Trans R Soc Trop Med Hyg 1935 Apr;28(6):645–8.

11. Rosenstein JL. Wound diphtheria in the newborn infant following circumcision. J Pediatr 1941 May;18(5):657–8.

12. Annunziato D, Goldman LM. Staphylococcal scalded skin syndrome: A complication of circumcision. Am J Dis Child 1978 Dec;132(12):1187–8.

Wiswell TE, Curtis J, Dobek AS, Zierdt CH. Staphylococcus aureus colonization after neonatal circumcision in relation to device used. J Pediatr 1991 Aug;119(2):302–4.

Enzenauer RW, Dotson CR, Leonard T Jr, Brown J 3rd, Pettett PG, Holton ME. Increased incidence of neonatal staphylococcal pyoderma in males. Mil Med 1984 Jul;149(7):408–10.

Enzenauer RW, Dotson CR, Leonard T Jr, Reuben L, Bass JW, Brown J III. Male predominance in persistent staphylococcal colonization and infection of the newborn. Hawaii Med J 1985 Oct;44(9):389–96.

Anday EK, Kobori J. Staphylococcal scalded skin syndrome: a complication of circumcision. Clin Pediatr (Phila) 1982 Jul;21(7):420.

13. Cleary TG, Kohl S. Overwhelming infection with group B beta-hemolytic streptococcus associated with circumcision. Pediatrics 1979 Sep;64(3):301–3.

14. Uwyyed K, Korman SH, Bar Oz B, Vromen A. Scrotal abscess with bacteremia caused by Salmonella group D after ritual circumcision. Pediatr Infect Dis J 1990 Jan;9(1):65–6.

Braun D. Neonatal bacteremia and circumcision. Pediatrics 1990 Jan;85(1):135–7.

15. Kirkpatrick BV, Eitzman DV. Neonatal septicemia after circumcision. Clin Pediatr (Phila) 1974 Sep;13(9):767–8.

Birrell R. A case against circumcision. Med J Aust 1965 Aug 28;2(9):393.

16. Scurlock JM, Pemberton PJ. Neonatal meningitis and circumcision. Med J Aust 1977 Mar 5;1(10):332–4.

17. Mahlberg FA, Rodermund OE, Muller RW. [A case of circumcision tuberculosis]. Hautarzt 1977 Aug;28(8):424–5.

18. Stranko J, Ryan ME, Bowman AM. Impetigo in newborn infants associated with a plastic bell clamp circumcision. Pediatr Infect Dis 1986 Sep–Oct;5(5):597–9.

19. Zafar AB, Butler RC, Reese DJ, Gaydos LA, Mennonna PA. Use of 0.3% triclosan (Bacti-Stat) to eradicate an outbreak of methicillin-resistant Staphylococcus aureus in a neonatal nursery. Am J Infect Control 1995 Jun;23(3):200–8.

Nelson JD, Dillon HC Jr, Howard JB. A prolonged nursery epidemic associated with a newly recognized type of group A streptococcus. J Pediatr 1976 Nov;89(5):792–6.

20. Dinari G, Haimov H, Geiffman M. Umbilical arteritis and phlebitis with scrotal abscess and peritonitis. J Pediatr Surg 1971 Apr;6(2):176.

21. Sauer LW. Fatal staphylococcus bronchopneumonia following ritual circumcision. Am J Obstetr Gynecol 1943 Oct;46(4):583.

Southby R. A case against circumcision. Med J Aust 1965 Aug 28;2(9):393.

22. Tammelleo AD. Nursing records "missing": spoilation of evidence. Case in point: Sweet v. Sisters of Providence in Wash. 881 P. 2d 304—AK (1994). Regan Rep Nurs Law 1994 Dec;35(7):2.

23. Editor. Medicolegal decisions: informed consent issue subject of case's remand. Am Med News 1997 Jul 7;49(25):38.

24. Johnson Flora Press Release. 8 March 2000.

25. Jim Sweet. Private correspondence. 25 June 1989. Cited in: Circumcision nightmare. The Truth Seeker 1989 Jul–Aug;1(3):52.

26. Woodside JR. Necrotizing fasciitis after neonatal circumcision. Am J Dis Child 1980 Mar:134(3):301–2.

Woodside JR. Circumcision disasters. Pediatrics 1980 May;65(5): 1053–4.

Bliss DP, Healey PJ, Waldhausen JHT. Necrotizing fasciitis after Plastibell circumcision. J Pediatr 1997 Sep;31(3):459–62.

Ngan JH, Mitchell M. Necrotizing fasciitis following neonatal circumcision. Conference presentation 15 February 1996, Department of Surgery at the Children's Hospital and Medical Center, University of Washington, Seattle, Washington. URL: http://www.infocirc.org/fourn.htm

Kaplan GW. Circumcision: an overview. Curr Probl Pediatr 1977 Mar;7(5):1–33.

Hamm WG, Kanthak FF. Gangrene of the penis following circumcision with high frequency current. South Med J 1949 Aug;42(8):657–9.

Thorek P, Egel P. Reconstruction of the penis with split-thickness skin graft: a case of gangrene following circumcision for acute balanitis. Plast Reconst Surg 1949 Sep;4(5):469–72.

Pinkham EW Jr, Stevenson AW Jr. Unusual reaction to local anesthesia: gangrene of the prepuce. US Armed Forces Med J 1958 Jan;9(1):120–2.

Rosefsky JB Jr. Glans necrosis as a complication of circumcision. Pediatrics 1967 May;39(5):774–6.

Sterenberg N, Golan J, Ben-Hur N. Necrosis of the glans penis following neonatal circumcision. Plast Reconstr Surg 1981 Aug;68(2):237–6.

Ahmed S, Shetty SD, Anandan N, Patil KP, Ibrahim AIA. Penile reconstruction following post-circumcision penile gangrene. Pediatr Surg Int 1994 Apr;9(4):295–6.

Kurel S. Iatrogenic penile gangrene: 10-year follow-up. Plast Reconst Surg 1995 Jan;95(1):210–1.

McGowan AJ Jr. A complication of circumcision. JAMA 1969 Mar 17;207(11);2104–5.

Stefan H. Reconstruction of the penis following necrosis from circumcision used high frequency cutting current. Sb Ved Pr Lek Fak Karlovy Univerzity Hradci Kralove 1992;35(5):449–54.

Stefan H. Reconstruction of the penis after necrosis due to circumcision burn. Eur J Pediatr Surg 1994 Feb;4(1):40–3.

Patel HI, Moriarty KP, Brisson PA, Feins NR. Genitourinary injuries in the newborn. J Pediatr Surg 2001 Jan;36(1):235–9.

Sussman SJ, Schiller RP, Shashikumar VL. Fournier's syndrome. Report of three cases and review of the literature. Am J Dis Child 1978 Dec;132(12):1189–91.

27. Adeyokunnu AA. Fournier's syndrome in infants. A review of cases from Ibadan, Nigeria. Clin Pediatr (Phila) 1983 Feb;22(2):101–3.

du Toit DF, Villet WT. Gangrene of the penis after circumcision: a report of 3 cases. S Afr Med J 1979 Mar 24;55(13):521–2.

Evbuomwan I, Aliu AS. Acute gangrene of the scrotum in a one month old child. Trop Geogr Med 1984 Sep;36(3):299–300.

28. Woodside JR. How to lessen risk of wound infection after circumcision. Mod Med 1980 Sep 30–Oct 15;48(16):93.

29. du Toit DF, Villet WT. Gangrene of the penis after circumcision: a report of 3 cases. S Afr Med J 1979 Mar 24;55(13):521–2.

30. Money J. Ablatio penis: normal male infant sex-reassigned as a girl. Arch Sex Behav 1975 Jan;4(1):65–71.

31. Sterenberg N, Golan J, Ben-Hur N. Necrosis of the glans penis following neonatal circumcision. Plast Reconst Surg 1981 Aug;68(2):237–6.

32. Foley JM. The unkindest cut of all. Fact 1966 Jul–Aug;3(4):2–9 [here, p. 6].

33. Stuehmer A. Balantis Xerotica Obliterans (post operationem) und ihre Beziehungen zur "Kraurosis Glandis et Praeputii Penis." Arch Derm Syph 1928;156:613–23.

Sprafke H. Balanitis Xerotica Obliterans Stühmer [A case of late postoperative, obliterative xerotic balanitis developing after circumcision]. Dermatologische Zeitschrift 1930;59(1):27–34.

Franks AG. Balanitis xerotica obliterans. J Urol 1946 Aug;56(2):243–5.

Potter B. Balanitis xerotica obliterans manifesting on the stump of amputated penis. Arch Dermatol 1959;79:473.

Weigand DA. Lichen sclerosus et atrophicus, multiple displastic keratosis and squamous cell carcinoma of the glans penis. J Dermatol Surg Oncol 1980 Jan;6(1):45–50.

Campus GV, Ena P, Scuderi N. Surgical treatment of balanitis xerotica obliterans. Plast Reconst Surg 1984 Apr;73(4):652–7.

Zungri E, Chechile G, Algaba F, Mallo N. Balanitis xerotica obliterans: surgical treatment. Eur Urol 1988;14(2):160–2.

Garat JM, Checile G, Algaba F, Santaularia JM. Balanitis xerotica obliterans in children. J Urol 1988 Aug;136(2):436–7.

Datta C, Dutta SR, Chaudhuri A. Histopathological and immunological studies in a cohort of balanitis xerotica obliterans. J Ind Med Assoc 1993 Jun;91(6):146–8.

34. Weigand DA. Lichen sclerosus et atrophicus, multiple displastic keratosis and squamous cell carcinoma of the glans penis. J Dermatol Surg Oncol 1980 Jan;6(1):45–50.

35. Amir J, Varsano I, Mimouni M. Circumcision and urinary tract infection in infants. Am J Dis Child 1986 Nov;140(11):1092.

Cohen HA, Drucker MM, Vainer S, Ashkenasi A, Amir J, Frydman M, Varsano I. Postcircumcision urinary tract infection. Clin Pediatr (Phila) 1992 Jun;31(6):322–4.

Goldman M, Barr J, Bistritzer T, Aladjem M. Urinary tract infection following ritual Jewish circumcision. Isr J Med Sci 1996 Nov; 32(11): 1098–102.

36. Ochsner MG. Acute urinary retention: causes and treatment. Postgrad Med 1982 Feb;71(2):221–6.

Craig JC, Grigor WG, Knight JF. Acute obstructive uropathy: a rare complication of circumcision. Eur J Pediatr 1994 May;153(5):369–71.

37. Horowitz J, Schussheim A, Scalettar HE. Letter: Abdominal distension following ritual circumcision. Pediatrics 1976 Apr;57(4):579.

38. Eason JD, McDonnell M, Clark G. Male ritual circumcision resulting in acute renal failure. Br Med J 1994 Sep 10;309(6955):660–1.

39. Berman W. Urinary retention due to ritual circumcision. Pediatrics 1975 Oct;56(4):621.

Frand M, Berant N, Brand N, Rotem Y. Complication of ritual circumcision in Israel. Pediatrics 1974 Oct;54(4):521.

Gee WF, Ansell JS. Neonatal circumcision: a ten-year overview: with comparison of the Gomco clamp and the Plastibell device. Pediatrics 1976 Dec;58(6):824–7.

40. Freud P. The ulcerated urethral meatus in male children. J Pediatr 1947 Aug;31(2):131–42.

Brennemann J. The ulcerated meatus in the circumcised child. Am J Dis Child 1921 Jan;21(1):38–47.

Mackenzie AR. Meatal ulceration following neonatal circumcision. Obstet Gynecol 1966 Aug;28(2):221–3.

Meyer HF. Meatal ulcer in the circumcised infant. Med Times 1971 Dec;99(12):77–8.

41. Mastin WM. Infantile circumcision: a cause of contraction of the external urethral meatus. Ann Anatomy Surg 1881 Jul–Dec;4:123–8.

Thompson AR. Stricture of the external urinary meatus. Lancet 1935 Jun 15;1(5833):1373–7.

Graves J. Pinpoint meatus: iatrogenic? Pediatrics 1968 May;41(5):1013.

Steg A, Allouch G. [Meatal stenosis and circumcision]. J Urol Nephrol Paris 1979 Oct–Nov;85(10–11):727–9.

Viville C, Weltzer J. [Iatrogenic stenosis of the male urethra: 50 cases]. J Urol (Paris) 1981;87(7):413–8.

Kunz HV. Circumcision and Meatotomy. Prim Care 1986 Sep;13(3): 513–5.

Frank JD, Pocock RD, Stower MJ. Urethral strictures in childhood. Br J Urol 1988 Dec;62(6):590–2.

Upadhyay V, Hammodat HM, Pease PW. Post circumcision meatal stenosis: 12 years' experience. N Z Med J 1998 Feb 27;111(1060):57–8.

42. Berry CD Jr, Cross RR Jr. Urethral meatal caliber in circumcised and uncircumcised males. J Dis Child 1956 Aug;92(2):152–6.

43. Persad R, Sharma S, McTavish J, Imber C, Mouriquand PDE. Clinical presentation and pathophysiology of meatal stenosis following circumcision. Br J Urol 1995 Jan;75(1):90–1.

44. Caldamone AA, Schulman S, Rabinowitz R. Outpatient pediatric urology. In: Gillenwater JY, Grayhack JT, Howards SS, Duckett JW (eds). Adult and Pediatric Urology 3rd ed. St. Louis: Mosby; 1996. vol. 3. pp. 2721–37.

45. Byars LT, Trier WC. Some complications of circumcision and their surgical repair. Arch Surg 1958 Mar;76(3):477–82.

Shulman J, Ben-Hur N, Neuman Z. Surgical complications of circumcision. Am J Dis Child 1964 Feb;107(2):149–54.

Johnson S. Peristent urethral fistula following circumcision: report of a case. US Naval Med Bull 1949 Jan;49(1):120–2.

Limaye RD, Hancock RA. Penile urethral fistula as a complication of circumcision. J Pediatr 1968 Jan;72(1):105–6.

Lackey JT, Mannion RA, Kerr JE. Urethral fistula following circumcision. JAMA 1968 Dec 2;206(10):2318.

Lackey JT, Mannion RA, Kerr JE. Subglanular urethral fistula from infant circumcision. J Ind State Med Assoc 1969 Nov;62(11):1305–6.

Shiraki IW. Congenital megalourethra with urethracutaneous fistula following circumcision: a case report. J Urol 1973 Apr:109(4):723–6.

Lau JTK, Ong GB. Subglanular urethral fistula following circumcision: repair by the advancement method. J Urol 1981 Nov;126(5):702–3.

Benchekroun A, Lakrissa A, Tazi A, Hafa D, Ouazzani N. [Urethral fistulas after circumcision: apropos of 15 cases]. Maroc Med 1981 Jun–Oct;3(2–3):715–8.

Tennenbaum SY, Palmer LS. Congenital urethrocutaneous fistulas. Urology 1994 Jan;43(1):98–9.

Colodny AH. Congenital urethrocutaneous fistulas. Urology 1994 Jul;44(1):149–50.

Baskin LS, Canning DA, Snyder HM 3rd, Duckett JW Jr. Surgical repair of urethral circumcision injuries. J Urol1997 Dec;158(6):2269–71.

46. McGowan AJ Jr. A complication of circumcision. JAMA 1969 Mar 17;207(11):2104–5.

47. Gee WF, Ansell JS. Neonatal circumcision: a ten-year overview: with comparison of the Gomco clamp and the Plastibell device. Pediatrics 1976 Dec;58(6):824–7.

Menahem S. Complications arising from ritual circumcision: pathogenesis and possible prevention. Isr J Med Sci 1981 Jan;17(1):45–8.

48. Shulman J, Ben-Hur N, Neuman Z. Surgical complications of circumcision. Am J Dis Child 1964 Feb;107(2):149–54.

49. Gairdner D. The fate of the foreskin: a study of circumcision. BMJ 1949 Dec 24;2(4642):1433–7.

50. Sara CA, Lowry CJ. A complication of circumcision and dorsal nerve block of the penis. Anaesth Intensive Care 1985 Feb;13(1):79–82.

Berens R, Pontus SP Jr. A complication associated with dorsal penile nerve block. Reg Anesth 1990 Nov–Dec;15(6):309–10.

Snellman LW, Stang HJ. Prospective evaluation of complications of dorsal penile nerve block for neonatal circumcision. Pediatrics 1995 May;95(5):705–8.

51. Tse S, Barrington K. Methemoglobinemia associated with prilocaine use in neonatal circumcision. Am J Perinatol 1995 Sep;12(5):331–2.

Couper RTL. Methaemoglobinaemia secondary to topical lignocaine/ prilocaine in a circumcised neonate. J Paediatr Child Health 2000 Aug;36(4): 406–7.

Arda IS, Özbek N, Akpek NE, Ersoy E. Toxic neonatal methaemoglobinaemia after prilocaine administration for circumcision. BJU Int 2000 May;85(9):1154.

Özbek N, Sarikayalar F. Toxic methaemoglobinaemia after circumcision. Eur J Pediatr 1993 Jan;152(1):80.

Mandel S. Methemoglobinemia following neonatal circumcision. JAMA 1989 Dec 3;261(5):702.

52. Fleiss PM, Douglass J. The case against neonatal circumcision. Brit Med J 1979 Sep 1;2(6189):554.

53. Lander J, Brady-Fryer B, Metcalfe JB, Nzarali S, Muttitt S. Comparison of ring block, dorsal penile nerve block, and topical anesthesia for neonatal circumcision: a randomized controlled trial. JAMA 1997 Dec 24–31;278(24):2157–62.

54. Auerbach MR, Scanlon JW. Recurrence of pneumothorax as a possible complication of elective circumcision. Am J Obstet Gynecol 1978 Nov;132(5):583.

55. Curtis JE. Circumcision complicated by pulmonary embolism. Nurs Mirror Midwives J 1971 Jun 18;132(25):28–30.

56. Ruff ML, Clarke TA, Harris JP, Bartels EK, Rosenzweig M. Myocardial injury following immediate postnatal circumcision. Am J Obstet Gynecol 1982 Dec;144(7):850–1.

57. Thompson HC, King LR, Knox E, Korones SB. Report of the ad hoc task force on circumcision. Pediatrics 1975 Oct;56(4):610–1.

58. Mor A, Eshel G, Aladjem M, Mundel G. Tachycardia and heart failure after circumcision. Arch Dis Child 1987 Jan;62(1):80–1.

59. Connelly KP, Shropshire LC, Salzberg A. Gastric rupture associated with prolonged crying in a newborn undergoing circumcision. Clin Pediatr (Phila) 1992 Sep;31(9):560–1.

60. Lee LD, Millar AJW. Ruptured bladder following circumcision using Plastibell device. Br J Urol 1990 Feb;65(2):216–7.

61. Arnon R, Zecharia A, Mimouni M, Merlob P. Unilateral leg cyanosis: an unusual complication of circumcision. Eur J Pediatr 1992 Sep;151(9):716.

62. Frand M, Berant N, Brand N, Rotem Y. Complication of ritual circumcision in Israel. Pediatrics 1974 Oct;54(4):521.

63. Stewart DH. The toad in the hole circumcision: a surgical bugbear. Bost Med Surg J 1924 Dec 25:191(26):1216–8.

Talarico RD, Jasaitis JE. Concealed penis: a complication of neonatal circumcision. J Urol 1973 Dec;110(6):732–3.

Trier WC, Drach GW. Concealed penis: another complication of circumcision. Am J Dis Child 1973 Feb;125(2):276–7.

Radhakrishnan J, Reyes HM. Penoplasty for buried penis secondary to "radical" circumcision. J Pediatr Surg 1984 Dec;19(6):629–31.

Kon M. A rare complication following circumcision: the concealed penis. J Urol 1983 Sep;130(3):573–4.

Donahoe PK, Keating MA. Preputial unfurling to correct the buried penis. J Pediatr Surg 1986 Dec;21(12):1055–7.

Maizels M, Zaontz M, Donovan J, Bushnick PN, Firlit CF. Surgical correction of the buried penis: description of a classification system and a technique to correct the disorder. J Urol 1986 Jul;136(1):268–73.

Shapiro SR. Surgical treatment of the "buried" penis. Urology 1987 Dec;30(6):554–9.

Horton CE, Vorstman B, Teasley D, Winslow B. Hidden penis release: adjunctive suprapubic lipectomy. Ann Plast Surg 1987 Aug;19(2):131–4.

Van der Zee JA, Hage JJ, Groen JM, Bouman FG. [A serious complication of ritual circumcision of a "buried" penis]. Ned Tijdschr Geneeskd 1991 Aug 31;135(35):1604–6.

Bergeson PS, Hopkin RJ, Bailey RB Jr, McGill LC, Piatt JP. The inconspicuous penis. Pediatrics 1993 Dec;92(6):794–9.

Alter GJ, Horton CE Jr; Horton CE. Buried penis as a contraindication for circumcision. J Am Coll Surg 1994 May;178(5):487–90.

64. Gracely-Kilgore KA. Penile adhesion: the hidden complication of circumcision. Nur Pract 1984 May;9(5):22–4.

65. Williams N, Kapila L. Complications of circumcision. Br J Surg 1993 Oct;1993;80:1231–6.

Brown JB. Restoration of the entire skin of the penis. Surg Gynecol Obstet 1937 Sep;65(3):362–5.

Wilson CL, Wilson MC. Plastic repair of the denuded penis. South Med J 1959 Mar;52(3):288–90.

Van Duyn J, Warr WS. Excessive penile skin loss from circumcision. J Med Assoc Ga 1962 Aug;51(8):394–6.

Sotolongo JR Jr; Hoffman S, Gribetz ME. Penile denudation injuries after circumcision. J Urol 1985 Jan;133(1):102–3.

Smey P. Re: Penile denudation injuries after circumcision. J Urol 1985 Dec;134(6):1220.

Orozco-Sanchez J, Neri-Vela R. [Total denudation of the penis in circumcision: description of a plastic technique for repair of the penis]. Bol Med Hosp Infant Mex 1991 Aug;48(8):565–9.

66. Kaplan GW. Circumcision: an overview. Curr Probl Pediatr 1977 Mar;7(5):1–33.

67. Kaplan GW. Circumcision: an overview. Curr Probl Pediatr 1977 Mar;7(5):1–33.

Shulman J, Ben-Hur N, Neuman Z. Surgical complications of circumcision. Am J Dis Child 1964 Feb;107(2):149–54.

68. Sathaye UV, Goswami AK, Sharma SK. Skin bridge—a complication of paediatric circumcision. Br J Urol 1990 Aug;66(2):214.

Ritchey ML, Bloom DA. Re: Skin bridge—a complication of paediatric circumcision. Br J Urol 1991 Sep;68(3):331.

Van Howe RS. Variability in penile appearance and penile findings: a prospective study. Br J Urol 1997 Nov;80(5):776–82.

Klauber GT, Boyle J. Preputial skin-bridging: complication of circumcision. Urology 1974 Jun;3(6):722–3.

Peters KM, Kass EJ. Electrosurgery for routine pediatric penile procedures. J Urol 1997 Apr;157(4):1453–5.

69. Kaplan GW. Circumcision: an overview. Curr Probl Pediatr 1977 Mar;7(5):1–33.

70. Datta NS, Zinner NR. Complications from Plastibell circumcision ring. Urology 1977 Jan;9(1):57–8.

Gee WF, Ansell JS. Neonatal circumcision: a ten-year overview: with comparison of the Gomco clamp and the Plastibell device. Pediatrics 1976 Dec;58(6):824–7.

Johnsonbaugh RE. Complication of a circumcision performed with a plastic disposable circumcision device: long-term follow-up. Am J Dis Child 1979 Apr;133(4):438.

Malo T, Bonforte RJ. Hazards of plastic bell circumcisions. Obstet Gynecol 1969 Jun;33(6):869.

Rubenstein MM, Bason WM. Complication of circumcision done with a plastic bell clamp. Am J Dis Child 1968 Oct;116(4):381–2.

Wright JE. Non-therapeutic circumcision. Med J Aust 1967 May 27;1(21):1083–6.

71. Warwick DJ, Dickson WA. Keloid of the penis after circumcision. Postgrad Med J 1993 Mar;69(809):236–7.

Gürünlüoğlu R, Bayramiçli M, Numanoğlu A. Keloid of the penis after circumcision. Br J Plast Surg 1996 Sep;49(6):425–6

Gürünlüoğlu R, Bayramiçli M, Dogan T, Numanoğlu A. Keloid after circumcision. Plast Reconst Surg 1999 Apr;103(5):1539–40.

Gürünlüoğlu R, Bayramiçli M, Numanoğlu A. Two patients with penile keloids: a review of the literature. Ann Plat Surg 1997 Dec;39(6):662–5.

Eldin US. Post-circumcision keloid: a case report. Annals of Burns and Fire Disasters 1999 Sep;12(3):174. URL: http://www.medbc.com/annals/review/vol 12/num 3/text/v12n3p174.htm

Michelowski R. Silica granuloma at the site of circumcision for phimosis: a case report. Dermatologica 1983;166(5):261–3.

Gürünlüoğlu R, Bayramiçli M, Dogan T, Numanoğlu A. Unusual complications of circumcision. Plast Reconst Surg 1999 Nov;104(6):1938–9.

72. Glover E. The "screening" function of traumatic memories. Int J Psychoanal 1929 Jan;10(1):90–3.

Hanash KA. Plastic reconstruction of partially amputated penis at circumcision. Urology 1976 Spe;18(3):291–3.

Stinson JM. Impotence and adult circumcision. J Nat Med Assoc 1973 Nov;65(2):161, 179.

Palmer JM, Link D. Impotence following anesthesia for electric circumcision. JAMA 1979 Jun 15;241(24):2635–6.

Stief CG, Thon WF, Djamilian M, et al., Transcutaneous registration of cavernous smooth muscle electrical activity: noninvasive diagnosis of neurogenic autonomic impotence. J Urol 1992 Jan;147(1):47–50.

73. Hanukoglu A, Danielli L, Katzir Z, Gorenstein A, Fried D. Serious complications of routine ritual circumcision in a neonate: hydroureteronephrosis, amputation of glans penis, and hyponatraemia. Eur J Pediatr 1995 Apr;154(4):314–5.

Gluckman GR, Stoller ML, Jacobs MM, Kogan BA. Newborn penile glans amputation during circumcision and successful reattachment. J Urol 1995 Mar;153(3):778–9.

Strimling BS. Partial amputation of glans penis during Mogen clamp circumcision. Pediatrics 1996 June;97(6):906–7.

Neulander E, Walfisch S, Kaneti J. Amputation of distal penile glans during neonatal ritual circumcision—a rare complication. Br J Urol 1996 Jun;77(6):924–5.

Sherman J, Borer JG, Horowitz M, Glassberg KI. Circumcision: successful glanular reconstruction and survival following amputation. J Urol1996 Aug;156(2):842–4.

Van Howe RS. Re: circumcision: successful glanular reconstruction and survival following traumatic amputation. J Urol 1997 Aug;158(2):550.

Coskunfirat OK, Sayilkan S, Velidedeoglu H. Glans and penile skin amputation as a complication of circumcision. Ann Plast Surg 1999 Oct;43(4):457.

74. Brown JB, Fryer MP. Surgical reconstruction of the penis. GP 1958 Apr;17(4):104–7.

Pearlman CK. Reconstruction following iatrogenic burn of the penis. J Pediatr Surg 1976 Feb;11(1):121–2.

Pearlman CK. Caution advised on electrocautery circumcisions. Urology 1982 Apr;19(4):453.

Stefan H. Reconstruction of the penis following necrosis from circumcision using high frequency cutting current. Sb Ved Pr Lek Fak Karlovy Univerzity Hradci Kralove 1992;35(5):449–54.

Gilbert DA, Jordan GH, Devine CJ Jr, Winslow BH, Schlossberg SM. Phallic construction in prepubertal and adolescent boys. J Urol 1993 Jun;149(6):1521–6.

Brimhall JB. Amputation of the penis following a unique method of preventing hemorrhage after circumcision. St Paul Med J 1902 Jul;4(7):490.

Lerner BL. Amputation of the penis as a complication of circumcision. Med Red Ann 1952 Sep;46(9):229–31.

Levitt SB, Smith RB, Ship AG. Iatrogenic microphallus secondary to circumcision. Urology 1976 Nov;8(5):472–4.

Izzidien AY. Successful replantation of a traumatically amputated penis in a neonate. J Ped Surg 1981 Apr;16(2):202–3.

Hanash KA. Plastic reconstruction of partially amputated penis at circumcision. Urology 1981 Sep;18(3):291–3.

Azmy A, Boddy SA, Ransley PG. Successful reconstruction following circumcision with diathermy. Br J Urol 1985 Oct;57(5):587–8.

Yilmaz AF, Sarikaya S, Yildiz S, Büyükalpelli R. Rare complication of circumcision: penile amputation and reattachment. Eur Urol 1993;23(3):423–4.

Audry G, Buis J, Vazquez MP, Gruner M. Amputation of penis after circumcision—penoplasty using expandable prosthesis. Eur J Pediatr Surg 1994 Feb;4(1):44–5.

Siegel-Itzkovich J. Baby's penis reattached after botched circumcision. BMJ 2000 Sep 2;321(7260):529.

Park JK, Min JK, Kim HJ. Reimplantation of an amputated penis in prepubertal boys. J Urol 2001 Feb;165(2):586–7.

75. Hanash KA. Plastic reconstruction of partially amputated penis at circumcision. Urology 1981 Sep;18(3):291–3.

Cetinkaya M, Saglam HS, Beyribey S. Two serious complications of circumcision. Case report. Scand J Urol Nephrol 1993;27(1):121–2.

76. Gilbert DA, Jordan GH, Devine CJ Jr, Winslow BH, Schlossberg SM. Phallic construction in prepubertal and adolescent boys. J Urol 1993 Jun;149(6):1521–6.

77. Money J. Ablatio penis: normal male infant sex-reassigned as a girl. Arch Sex Behavior 1975 Jan;4(1):65–71.

Gearhart JP, Rock JA. Total ablation of the penis after circumcision with electrocautery: a method of management and long-term followup. J Urol 1989 Sep;142(3):799–801.

Diamond M, Sigmundson HK. Sex reassignment at birth: long-term review and clinical implications. Arch Pediatr Adolesc Med 1997 Mar;151(3): 298–304.

Bradley SJ, Oliver GD, Chernick AB, Zuker KJ. Experiment of nurture: ablatio penis at 2 months, sex reassignment at 7 months, and a psychosexual follow-up in young adulthood. Pediatrics 1998 Jul;102(1):e9.

78. Schepers D. Pioneer leaves his mark on pediatric education: Gellis' legacy rooted in students, colleagues, family. AAP News 1997 Feb;13(2):26.

79. Gellis SS. Circumcision. Am J Dis Child 1978 Dec;132(12):1168–9.

80. Gellis SS. Circumcision. Am J Dis Child 1979 Oct;133(10):1079–80.

81. McCarty JF. Reaction to anesthesia killed baby boy, report says. Cleveland Plain Dealer (21 October 1998): URL: http://www.cleveland. com/news/pdnews/metro/crainbow.phtml

82. Scurlock JM, Pemberton PJ. Neonatal meningitis and circumcision. Med J Aust 1977 Mar 5;1(10):332–4.

83. Cleary TG, Kohl S. Overwhelming infection with group B beta-hemolytic streptococcus associated with circumcision. Pediatrics 1979 Sep;64(3):301–3.

84. Baker RL. Newborn male circumcision: needless and dangerous. Sexual Medicine Today 1979 Nov;3(11):35–6.

85. Grimes D. Routine circumcision of the newborn infant: a reappraisal. Am J Obstet Gynecol 1978 Jan 15;130(2):125–9.

86. Racher P. Grand jury to probe death of baby after circumcision. Des Moines Register. (20 November 1982):3A.

Associated Press. Boy in coma most of his 6 years dies. The State (Columbia, South Carolina) (10 July 1992):5B.

Rogers P, Wallace R. Infant bleeds to death after being circumcised. Miami Herald (26 June 1993):B1–B2.

Lum L, SoRelle R. Boy's autopsy results expected: five-year-old lapsed into coma following circumcision. Houston Chronicle (28 July 1995):28A.

Associated Press. Circumcision that didn't heal kills boy: the boy's circumcision wasn't healing properly. News Net 5. (20 October 1998): URL: http://www.newsnet5.com/news/stories/news-981020-051123.html

Foley JM. The unkindest cut of all. Fact 1966 Jul;3(4):2–9.

87. Rogers P, Wallace R. Infant bleeds to death after being circumcised. Miami Herald (26 June 1993):B1–B2.

88. Racher P. Grand jury to probe death of baby after circumcision. Des Moines Register (20 November 1982):3A.

89. Lum L, SoRelle R. Boy's autopsy results expected: five-year-old lapsed into coma following circumcision. Houston Chronicle (28 July 1995):28A.

90. Associated Press. Circumcision that didn't heal kills boy: the boy's circumcision wasn't healing properly. News Net 5. (20 October 1998): URL: http://www.newsnet5.com/news/stories/news-981020-051123.html

91. Menage J. Post traumatic stress disorder after genital medical procedures. In: Denniston GC, Hodges FM, Milos MF (eds). Male and Female Circumcision: Medical, Legal, and Ethical Considerations in Pediatrics Practice. New York: Kluwer Academic/Plenum Publishers; 1999. pp. 215–9.

92. Rhinehart J. Neonatal circumcision reconsidered. Transactional Analysis Journal 1999 Jul;29(3):215–21.

Bensley GA, Boyle GJ. Physical, sexual, and psychological effects of infant circumcision: an exploratory survey. In: Denniston GC, Hodges FM, Milos MF (eds). Understanding Circumcision: A Multi-Disciplinary Approach to a Multi-Dimensional Problem. New York: Kluwer Academic/Plenum Publishers; 2001. pp. 207–39.

Gemmell T, Boyle GJ. Neonatal circumcision: its long-term harmful effects. In: Denniston GC, Hodges FM, Milos MF (eds). Understanding Circumcision: A Multi-Disciplinary Approach to a Multi-Dimensional

Problem. New York: Kluwer Academic/Plenum Publishers; 2001. pp. 241–52.

Ramos, S, Boyle GJ. Ritual and medical circumcision among Filipino boys: evidence of post-traumatic stress disorder. In: Denniston GC, Hodges FM, Milos MF (eds). Understanding Circumcision: A Multi-Disciplinary Approach to a Multi-Dimensional Problem. New York: Kluwer Academic/ Plenum Publishers; 2001. pp. 253–70.

93. Menage J. Post traumatic stress disorder after genital medical procedures. In: Denniston GC, Hodges FM, Milos MF (eds). Male and Female Circumcision: Medical, Legal, and Ethical Considerations in Pediatrics Practice. New York: Kluwer Academic/Plenum Publishers; 1999. pp. 215–9.

94. Wiswell TE. Do you favor . . . routine neonatal circumcision? Yes. Postgrad Med 1988 Oct;84(5):98, 100, 102, 104, passim.

95. Gluckman GR, Stoller ML, Jacobs MM, Kogan BA. Newborn penile glans amputation during circumcision and successful reattachment. J Urol 1995 Mar;153(3):778–9.

Chapter 5: Disadvantages of Circumcision

1. Sorger L. To ACOG: stop circumcisions. Ob Gyn News 1994 Nov 1;29(21):8.

2. Halata Z, Munger BL. The neuroanatomical basis for the protopathic sensibility of the human glans penis. Brain Res 1986 Apr 23;371(2):205–30.

Chapter 6: Circumcision in Religion

1. Wine ST. Circumcision. Humanistic Judaism 1988 Summer;16(3): 4–8.

2. Gospel of Thomas 53. In: Schneemelcher W, Wilson R. McL (eds). 2 vols. New Testament Apocrypha. Cambridge: J. Clarke & Co; Louisville, Ky: Westminster/John Knox Press. 1991–1992. 1, p. 125.

3. Esra 5:30–31. The Fifth and Sixth Books of Esra. Esra 5:30–31. The Fifth and Sixth Books of Esra. In: Schneemelcher W, Wilson R. McL (eds). 2 vols. New Testament Apocrypha. Cambridge: J. Clarke & Co; Louisville, Ky: Westminster/John Knox Press. 1991–1992. vol. 2, pp. 643–4.

4. Paulus, Sententiae 5:22:3–4. In: Linder A. (ed). The Jews in Roman Imperial Legislation. Detroit: Wayne State University Press; 1987. pp. 117–20.

5. Collectio Tripartita, book 1: from the codex. Title 9, Translation 70.

Linder A (ed). The Jews in the Legal Sources of the Early Middle Ages. Detroit: Wayne State University Press; 1997. p. 49.

6. The canons of the holy and altogether august apostles. In: Percival HR (ed). The Seven Ecumenical Councils of the Undivided Church. vol. 14 of: A Select Library of Nicene and Post-Nicene Fathers of the Christian Church. 2nd series. New York: Charles Scribner's Sons; 1900. p. 595.

7. St. Augustine. Reply to Faustus the Manichaean. Book XIX. Paragraph 9. In: Dods M (ed). The Works of Aurelius Augustine, Bishop of Hippo. Edinburgh: T. & T. Clark. 1872. vol. 15, p. 334.

8. St. Cyril. The Catechetical Lectures. In: Schaff P. Wace H (eds). A Select Library of Nicene and Post-Nicene Fathers of the Christian Church. Second Series. 14 vols. New York: The Christian Literature Company. 1894. vol. 7, p. 30.

9. St. Jerome. Epistola XIX: De vera circumcisione. In: Migne JP (ed). S. Eusebii Hieronymi, Opera Omnia. Patrologiae cursus completes. Paris: n.p.; 1846. vol. 11, pp. 188–210.

10. St. John Chrysostom. Discourses Against Judaizing Christians. Translated by Paul W. Harkins. Washington, DC: The Catholic University of America Press; 1979.

11. John of Damascus. Exposition of the Orthodox Faith. Chapter XXV. Concerning the Circumcision. In: Watson EW, Pullan L (eds). A Select Library of Nicene and Post-Nicene Fathers of the Christian Church. 2nd series. 14 vols. New York: The Christian Literature Company. 1894. vol. 9, p. 97.

12. St. Justin Martyr. Dialogue with Trypho. In: Falls TB (ed). Writings of Saint Justin Martyr. New York: Christian Heritage; 1948. pp. 147–368 [here, pp. 171–84, 212–9].

13. Lactantius. The Divine Institutes, XVII. Of the superstitions of the Jews, and their hatred against Jesus. In: Roberts A, Donaldson J (eds). The Ante-Nicene Fathers. 10 vols. Buffalo: The Christian Literature Company; 1886. vol. 7, pp. 118–9.

14. Origen. De Principiis, 4.3. In: Butterworth GW (ed). Origen on First Principles. London: Society for Promoting Christian Knowledge. 1936. p. 293.

15. Tertullian. Adversus Iudaeos II, 13-III. In: Quinti Septimi Florentis Tertulliani Opera, Pars II. Opera Montantistica. Turnholti: Typographi Brepols; 1954. pp. 1344–9.

16. St. Ambrose. Ambrose to Constantius. In: Beyenka MM (trans). Saint Ambrose Letters. New York: Fathers of the Church. 1954. pp. 90–100.

St. Ambrose. Ambrose to Horontianus. In: Beyenka MM (trans). Saint Ambrose Letters. New York: Fathers of the Church. 1954. pp. 251–4.

17. Origen. Against Celsus 22. In: The Ante-Nicene Fathers. 10 vols. Buffalo: The Christian Literature Company; 1886. vol. 4, p. 405.

18. St. Ambrose. Ambrose to Clementianus. In: Beyenka MM (trans). Saint Ambrose Letters. New York: Fathers of the Church. 1954. pp. 405–9 [here, p. 407].

19. Grayzel S. The Church and the Jews in the XIIth Century. vol. 2, ed. K. R. Stow. Detroit, MI: Wayne State University Press; 1989. pp. 246–7.

Linder A (ed). The Jews in the Legal Sources of the Early Middle Ages. Detroit: Wayne State University Press; 1997. pp. 28, 35, 38, 49, 52–8, 73, 84, 87, 104, 106, 113–9, 127, 133–6, 141–4, 147, 155–8, 170, 172, 213, 214, 226, 233, 238, 242–4, 248–53, 257, 260, 264, 268, 270, 274, 278, 285, 290, 295, 314, 351, 406, 409, 413, 416, 485, 488, 499, 519, 543, 576–7, 583, 587, 612–3, 617, 619–20, 636, 656, 658, 669, 670, 679.

20. See: Pelikan J, Oswald HC, Grimm HJ, Lehmann HT (eds). Luther's Works. 55 vols. Philadelphia: Fortress Press; 1971. vol. 2, p. 361; vol. 47, pp. 88, 152–9; vol. 54, p. 239.

21. Moroni 8:8. The Book of Mormon. Translated by Joseph Smith. First published in 1830. Salt Lake City: The Church of Jesus Christ of Latter-Day Saints; 1921. p. 516.

22. Section 74:2–7. Doctrine and Covenants. Salt Lake City: Deseret News Company; 1880. pp. 260–1.

23. Rosenberg D, Bloom H (trans and eds). The Book of J. New York: Grove Weidenfeld; 1990. p. 79.

24. Hoffman LA. Covenant of Blood: Circumcision and Gender in Rabbinic Judaism. Chicago & London: University of Chicago Press; 1996.

25. Mishnah. Shabbath 19:1–6. In: The Mishnah. Translated by Herbert Danby. Oxford: Oxford University Press; 1933. pp. 116–7.

26. Talmud of Babylon. Shabbat 133B. In: The Talmud of Babylonia: An American Translation. Translated by Jacob Neusner. Number 275. Volume II.E: Shabbat Chapters 18–24. Program in Judaic Studies, Brown University. Atlanta: Scholars Press; 1993. p. 45.

27. Romberg HC. Bris Milah: A Book About the Jewish Ritual of Circumcision. Jerusalem/New York: Feldheim Publishers; 1982.

28. Shamash J. My son at the cutting edge. The Independent (London) (17 December 1998): p. R8 (The Thursday Review).

29. Hofmokl. Letter from Vienna: Tuberculosis communicated in the rite of circumcision. New York Medical Journal 1886 Aug 21;44:213–4.

Elsenberg A. Inoculation of tuberculosis by circumcision. BMJ 1887 Mar 5;1(1366):525.

Lehmann E. Lehmann on a mode of inoculative tuberculosis in man. London Medical Record 1887 Mar 15:15(3):128.

Shrady GF. Tuberculosis from circumcision. Medical Record 1887 Mar 26;31(13):355.

Eve FS. Communication of tuberculosis by ritual circumcision. Lancet 1888 Jan 28;1(3361):170–1.

Meyer W. Ein Fall von Impftuberkulose infolge ritueller Zirkumzision. New-Yorker Medizinische Presse 1887 Jun;4(1):1–7.

Koltzoff AI. An epidemic of cutaneous tuberculosis spread through ritual circumcision. British Journal of Dermatology 1890 Oct;2(10):323.

Kinnicutt FP. Tuberculosis infection by circumcision. Medical Record 1893 Mar 4;43(9):285.

Ware MW. A case of inoculation tuberculosis after circumcision. New York Medical Journal 1898 Feb 26;67:287–8.

Neumann. Tuberculosis inoculated by circumcision. American Journal of Obstetrics and Diseases of Women and Children 1899 Apr;39(4):575.

Bernhardt R. Tuberculosis as a sequel of ritual circumcision. New York Medical Journal 1901 Dec 21;74:1176.

Welt-Kakels S. Inoculation tuberculosis following ritual circumcision. American Journal of Obstetrics and Diseases of Women and Children 1909 Apr;69(4):1073–8.

Arluck IM, Winocouroff IJ. Tuberculosis acquired at circumcision. JAMA 1912 Jun 15;58(24):1885.

Holt LE. Tuberculosis acquired through ritual circumcision. JAMA 1913 Jul 12;61(2):99–102.

30. Taylor RW. On the question of the transmission of syphilitic contagion in the rite of circumcision. New York Medical Journal 1873 Dec;18(6): 561–82.

Lubelski G. Note sur la propagation de la syphilis par la circoncision des enfants Israélies en Pologne. Revue d'Hygiène et de Police Sanitaire 1881 Jul;3:377–9.

Lubelski. On the propagation of syphilis in Poland by the circumcision of Jewish children. London Medical Record 1882 Jun 15;10(6):244.

Kédotoff A. Transmission de la syphilis par la circoncision pratiquée d'après le procédé hébraïque. Annales de Dermatologie et Syphiliographie 1884 Sep 25–Oct 25;5(9–10):526–9.

Popper, Kapose, Grünfeld, Lang, Hock, Neumann. Syphilis à la suite de la circoncision. Gazette Hebdomadaire de Médecine et de Chirurgie 1896 Mar 19;43(23):276.

Morrow PA. A case of syphilis from ritual circumcision. Journal of Cutaneous Diseases Including Syphilis 1903 May;21(5):235.

31. Hasbrouck E. Circumcision, erysipelas, diphtheria and death. North American Journal of Homœopathy 1895 Aug;43(8):470–4.

Beatty RP. Diphtheria of the glans penis following circumcision. BMJ 1907 Nov 30;2(2448):1582.

Kolmer JA. Diphtheroid bacilli of the penis, with report of 2 cases of diphtheria following circumcision. Archives of Pediatrics 1912 Feb;29(2):94–101.

Borovsky MP. Diphtheria of the penis. JAMA 1935 Apr 20;104(16):1399–401.

32. See the short discussion of this history in: Gilman SL. Freud, Race, and Gender. Princeton: Princeton University Press; 1993. pp. 66–9.

33. Rubin LG, Lanzkowsky P. Cutaneous neonatal herpes simplex infection associated with ritual circumcision. Pediatr Infect Dis J 2000 Mar;19(3):266–8.

34. Romberg HC. Bris Milah: A Book About the Jewish Ritual of Circumcision. Jerusalem/New York: Feldheim Publishers; 1982. pp. 57–8.

35. Friedländer M, trans. The Guide of the Perplexed of Maimonides. 3 parts. New York: Hebrew Publishing Co.; 1881. part III. p. 267.

36. Glick LB. Jewish circumcision: an enigma in historical perspective. In: Denniston GC, Hodges FM, Milos FM (eds). Understanding Circumcision: A Multi-Disciplinary Approach to a Multi-Faceted Problem. New York and London: Kluwer Academic/Plenum Publishers; 2001. pp. 19–54.

37. Geiger A. Abraham Geigers Nachgelassene Schriften. vol. 5. Berlin: Louis Gerschel; 1878. (Letter to L. Zunz, March 19, 1845), p. 181. Translation by Leonard B. Glick with assistance from Anne Spier-Mazor.

38. Elon A. Herzl. New York: Holt, Rinehart and Winston; 1975. p. 93.

39. Rothenberg J. The Jewish Religion in the Soviet Union. New York: KTAV Publishing House; 1971. pp. 141–67.

Rothenberg J. Jewish religion in the Soviet Union. In: Kochan L (ed). Jewish Religion in the Soviet Union. London: Oxford University Press; 1970. p. 184.

Gitelman Z. The communist party and Soviet Jewry: the early years. In: Marshall RH Jr (ed). Aspects of Religion in the Soviet Union: 1917–1967. Chicago: University of Chicago Press; 1971. p. 332.

Rothenberg J. The Jewish religion in the Soviet Union since World War II. In: Marshall RH Jr (ed). Aspects of Religion in the Soviet Union: 1917–1967. Chicago: University of Chicago Press; 1971. p. 346.

Kolarz W. Religion in the Soviet Union. London: Macmillan; 1966. pp. 347, 355, 442.

40. Goodman J. Jewish circumcision: an alternative perspective. BJU Int 1999 Jan;83:22–7.

41. Goldman R. Circumcision: The Hidden Trauma: How an American Cultural Practice Affects Infants and Ultimately Us All. Boston: Vanguard Publications; 1997.

Goldman R. The psychological impact of circumcision. BJU Int 1999 Jan;83(Suppl 1):93–102.

42. Goldman R. Questioning Circumcision: A Jewish Perspective. Boston: Vanguard Publications; 1998. pp. 95–108.

43. Goldman R. Questioning Circumcision: A Jewish Perspective. Boston: Vanguard Publications; 1998.

44. Aldeeb Abu-Sahlieh, SA. Jehovah, his cousin Allah, and sexual mutilations. In: Denniston GC, Milos MF (eds). Sexual Mutilations: A Human Tragedy. New York: Plenum Press; 1997. pp. 41–62.

45. The Geography of Strabo. Jones HL, trans. 8 vols. Cambridge: Harvard University Press; 1966. vol. 7. pp. 315, 323, 339.

46. Foreign Department Editor. Circumcision at Tangiers. Lancet 1851 Mar 1;1(1435):241.

47. Crowley IP, Kesner KM. Ritual circumcision (umkhwetha) amongst the Xhosa of the Ciskei. Br J Urol 1990 Sep;66(3):318–21.

Malherbe WDF. Injuries to the skin of the male external genitalia in Southern Africa. S Afr Med J 1975 Feb 1;49(5):147–52.

Sibusiso Bubesi. Children kidnapped and mutilated: boy threatened with death after investigation of circumcision camps. Sunday Times (Cape Town), (14 March 1999). URL: p. http://www.suntimes.co.za/1999/03/14/news/news03.htm

Editor. Ten die after circumcisions. Independent (London), (22 July 1999):p. 12.

McGreal C. Botched circumcision kills boys. Guardian (London), (7 January 2000):p. 16.

48. Mkokeli S. Traditional leaders vow to defy traditional circumcision act. East Cape News. (October 26, 2001). URL: http://allafrica.com/stories/200110260368.html

49. Ghanem AN. Religious circumcision: a Moslem view. BJU Int 1999 Sep;84(4):543.

50. Chabukswar YV. Barbaric method of circumcision amongst some Arab tribes of Yemen. Indian Medical Gazette 1921 Feb;56(2):48–9.

51. Bissada NK, Morcos RR, El-Senoussi M. Post-circumcision carcinoma of the penis. I. Clinical aspects. J Urol 1986 Feb;135(2):283–5.

Koriech OM. Penile shaft carcinoma in pubic circumcision. Br J Urol 1987 Jul;60(1):77.

52. Yüksel, Edip. Circumcision. 2001. URL: http://www.quran.org/khatne.htm

Chapter 7: The History of Circumcision

1. Clarke AC. Cruel cut. New Scientist 2000 Jan 15; 165(2221):51.

2. DeMeo J. The geography of male and female genital mutilations. In: Denniston GC, Milos MF (eds). Sexual Mutilations: A Human Tragedy. New York: Plenum Press; 1997. pp. 1–15.

3. Strachey J, Freud A, et al. (eds). The Standard Edition of the Complete Psychological Works of Sigmund Freud. 24 vols. London: The Hogarth Press and the Institute of Psycho-Analysis; 1953–1974. vol. 10, p. 36; vol. 11, pp. 95–96, n. 3; vol. 13, p. 153; vol. 15, pp. 164–5; vol. 17, p. 86; vol. 22, pp. 86–7, vol. 23, pp. 91, 190, n. 1.

4. Hodges FM. The ideal prepuce in ancient Greece and Rome: male genital aesthetics and their relation to lipodermos, circumcision, foreskin restoration, and the kynodesmē. Bull Hist Med 2001 Fall;75(3):375–405.

5. Strabo. Geography 16.2.37. In: Jones HL (trans). The Geography of Strabo. 8 vols. Cambridge: Harvard University Press; 1917–1932. vol. 7, p. 285.

Diodorus Siculus. The Library of History 1.28. In: Oldfather CH (trans). Diodorus of Sicily. 12 vols. Cambridge: Harvard University Press; 1933–1967. vol. 1, p. 91.

6. Strabo. Geography 16.4.5. In: Jones HL (trans). The Geography of Strabo. 8 vols. Cambridge: Harvard University Press; 1917–1932. vol. 7, p. 315, 323.

7. Diodorus Siculus. The Library of History 3.32. In: Oldfather CH (trans). Diodorus of Sicily. 12 vols. Cambridge: Harvard University Press; 1933–1967. vol. 2, p. 173.

8. I Maccabees, 1:15.

9. Linder A. (ed). The Jews in Roman Imperial Legislation. Detroit: Wayne State University Press; 1987. pp. 100, 117–20.

10. Linder A. (ed). The Jews in the Legal Sources of the Early Middle Ages. Detroit: Wayne State University Press; 1997. pp. 28, 35, 38, 49, 52–58, 73, 84, 87, 104, 106, 113–9, 127, 133–6, 138–44, 147, 155–8, 170, 172, 213, 214, 226, 233, 238, 242–4, 248–53, 257, 260, 264, 268, 270, 274, 278, 285, 290, 295, 314, 351, 406, 409, 413, 416, 485, 488, 499, 519, 543, 576–7, 583, 587, 612–3, 617, 619–20, 636, 656, 658, 669, 670, 679.

11. Gollaher DL. From ritual to science: the medical transformation of circumcision in America. J Soc Hist 1994 Fall;28(1):5–36.

Gollaher DL. Circumcision: A History of the World's Most Controversial Surgery. New York: Basic Books; 2000.

12. Moses MJ. The value of circumcision as a hygienic and therapeutic measure. New York Medical Journal 1871 Nov;14(4):368–74.

13. Money A. Treatment of Disease in Children. Philadelphia: P. Blakiston; 1887. p. 421.

14. Hodges FM. A short history of the institutionalization of involuntary sexual mutilation in the United States. In: Denniston GC, Milos FM (eds). Sexual Mutilations: A Human Tragedy. New York: Plenum Press; 1997. pp. 17–40.

15. Hutchinson J. On circumcision as preventive of masturbation. Archives of Surgery 1891 Jan;2(7):267–8.

16. Hodges FM. A short history of the institutionalization of involuntary sexual mutilation in the United States. In: Denniston GC, Milos FM (eds). Sexual Mutilations: A Human Tragedy. New York: Plenum Press; 1997. pp. 17–40.

17. Robinson WJ. Circumcision and masturbation. Medical World 1915 Oct;33(10):390.

18. Remondino PC. History of Circumcision from the Earliest Times to the Present. Philadelphia: F. A. Davis; 1891. pp. 161–82.

19. Remondino PC. History of Circumcision from the Earliest Times to the Present. Philadelphia: F. A. Davis; 1891.

20. Remondino PC. Circumcision and its opponents. American Journal of Dermatology and Genito-Urinary Diseases 1902 Mar;6(2):65–73 [here, p. 66].

21. Remondino PC. History of Circumcision from the Earliest Times to the Present. Philadelphia: F. A. Davis; 1891. p. 290.

22. Remondino PC. Negro rapes and their social problems. National Popular Review 1894 Jan;4(1):3–6 [here, pp. 3–4].

23. Remondino PC. Circumcision and its opponents. American Journal of Dermatology and Genito-Urinary Diseases 1902 Mar;6(2):65–73.

24. Wolbarst AL. Universal circumcision as a sanitary measure. JAMA 1914 Jan 10;62(2):92–7.

25. Hofmokl. Letter from Vienna: tuberculosis communicated in the rite of circumcision. New York Medical Journal 1886 Aug 21;44:213–4.

Elsenberg A. Inoculation of tuberculosis by circumcision. BMJ 1887 Mar 5;1(1366):525.

Lehman E. Lehmann on a mode of inoculative tuberculosis in man. London Medical Record 1887 Mar 15;15(3):128.

Shrady GF. Tuberculosis from circumcision. Medical Record 1887 Mar 26:31(13):355.

Eve FS. Communication of tuberculosis by ritual circumcision. Lancet 1888 Jan 28;1(3361):170–1.

Meyer W. Ein fall von Impftuberkulose infolge ritueller Zirkumzision. New-Yorker Medizinische Presse 1887;4(1):1–7.

Koltzoff AI. An epidemic of cutaneous tuberculosis spread through ritual circumcision. British Journal of Dermatology 1890 Oct;2(10):323.

Kinnicutt FP. Tuberculosis infection by circumcision. Medical Record 1893 Mar 4;43(9):285.

Ware MW. A case of inoculation tuberculosis after circumcision. New York Medical Journal 1898 Feb 26;67:287–8.

Neumann. Tuberculosis inoculated by circumcision. American Journal of Obstetrics and Diseases of Women and Children 1899 Apr;39(4):575.

Bernhardt R. Tuberculosis as a sequel of ritual circumcision. New York Medical Journal 1901 Dec 21;74:1176.

Welt-Kakels S. Inoculation tuberculosis following ritual circumcision. American Journal of Obstetrics and Diseases of Women and Children 1909 Apr;69(4):1073–8.

Arluck IM, Winocouroff IJ. Tuberculosis acquired at circumcision. JAMA 1912 Jun 15;58(24):1885.

Holt LE. Tuberculosis acquired through ritual circumcision. JAMA 1913 Jul 12;61(2):99–102.

Taylor RW. On the question of the transmission of syphilitic contagion in the rite of circumcision. New York Medical Journal 1873 Dec;18(6): 561–82.

Lubelski G. Note sur la propagation de la syphilis par la circoncision des enfants Israélites en Pologne. Revue d'Hygiène et de Police Sanitaire 1881 Jul;3:377–9.

Lubelski. On the propagation of syphilis in Poland by the circumcision of Jewish children. London Medical Record 1882 Jun 15;10(6):244.

Kédotoff A. Transmission de la syphilis par la circoncision pratiquée d'après le procédé hébraïque. Annales de Dermatologie et Syphiliographie 1884 Sep 25–Oct 25;5(9–10):526–9.

Popper, Kapose, Grünfeld, Lang, Hock, Neumann. Syphilis à la suite de la circoncision. Gazette Hebdomadaire de Médecine et de Chirurgie 1896 Mar 19;43(23):276.

Morrow PA. A case of syphilis from ritual circumcision. Journal of Cutaneous Diseases Including Syphilis 1903 May;21(5):235.

Hasbrouck E. Circumcision, erysipelas, diphtheria and death. North American Journal of Homœopathy 1895 Aug;43(8):470–4.

Beatty RP. Diphtheria of the glans penis following circumcision. BMJ 1907 Nov 30;2(2448):1582.

Kolmer JA. Diphtheroid bacilli of the penis, with report of 2 cases of diphtheria following circumcision. Archives of Pediatrics 1912 Feb;29(2):94–101.

Borovsky MP. Diphtheria of the penis. JAMA 1935 Apr 20;104(16): 1399–401.

26. Wolbarst AL. Persistent masturbation. JAMA 1932 Jul 9;99(2): 154–5.

27. Guttmacher AF. Should the baby be circumcised? Parents' Magazine 1941 Sep;16(9):26,76–8.

28. Fishbein M. Sex hygiene. In: Fishbein M (ed). Modern Home Medical Adviser. Garden City, New York: Doubleday & Company; 1969. p. 119.

29. Fishbein M. Sex hygiene. In: Fishbein M (ed). Modern Home Medical Adviser. Garden City, New York: Doubleday & Company; 1969. pp. 90, 119.

30. Fishbein M. Sex hygiene. In: Fishbein M (ed). Modern Home Medical Adviser. Garden City, New York: Doubleday & Company; 1969. pp. 90.

31. Gerber ML. Some practical aspects of circumcision. US Naval Med Bull 1944 May;42(5):1147–9.

32. Gerber ML. Some practical aspects of circumcision. US Naval Med Bull 1944 May;42(5):1147–9.

33. Ravich A. The relationship of circumcision to cancer of the prostate. J Urol 1942 Sep;48(3):298–9.

34. Ravich A, Ravich RA. Prophylaxis of cancer of the prostate, penis, and cervix by circumcision. N Y State J Med 1951 Jun;51(12):1519–20.

35. Ravich A. Viral carcinogenesis in venereally susceptible organs. Cancer 1971 Jun;27(6):1493–6.

36. Ravich A. Preventing V.D. and Cancer by Circumcision. New York: Philosophical Library; 1973. pp. 33–6, 152, 157.

37. Ravich A. The Relationship of Circumcision to Cancer of the Prostate. J Urol 1942 Sep;48(3):298–9.

Ravich A. Preventing V.D. and Cancer by Circumcision. New York: Philosophical Library; 1973.

38. Reddy G, Baruah IKSM. Carcinogenic action of human smegma. Arch Path 1963 Apr;75(4):414–20.

39. Rothenberg RE (ed). The New Illustrated Medical Encyclopedia for Home Use: A Practical Guide to Good Health. 4 vols. New York: Abradale Press; 1959. vol. 3, pp. 823–6.

40. Spock B. The Commonsense Book of Baby and Child Care. New York: Duell, Sloan & Pearce; 1946.

41. Spock B. The Commonsense Book of Baby and Child Care. New York: Duell, Sloan & Pearce; 1957. p. 155.

42. Spock B, Rothenberg MB. Dr. Spock's Baby and Child Care. New York: Pocket Books; 1992. pp. 225–7.

43. Miller RL, Snyder DC. Immediate circumcision of the newborn male. Am J Obstet Gynecol 1953 Jan;65(1):1–11.

44. Campbell MF. The male genital tract and the female urethra. In: Campbell MF, Harrison JH (eds). Urology. 3rd ed. 3 vols. Philadelphia: WB Saunders; 1970. vol. 2, pp. 1834–87 [here, p. 1836].

45. Campbell MF. The male genital tract and the female urethra. In: Campbell MF, Harrison JH (eds). Urology. 3rd ed. 3 vols. Philadelphia: WB Saunders; 1970. vol. 2, pp. 1834–87 [here, p. 1836].

46. Van J, Kotulak R. Circumcision: expensive and unnecessary ritual. Chicago Tribune (6 October 1980): pp. 1, 11.

47. Weiss GN. Prophylactic neonatal surgery and infectious diseases. Pediatr Infect Dis J 1997 Aug;16(8):727–34.

48. Fink AJ. Circumcision and sand. J R Soc Med 1991 Nov;84(11): 696.

49. Committee on Fetus and Newborn. Circumcision. In: Hospital Care of Newborn Infants. 5th ed. Evanston, Ill: American Academy of Pediatrics; 1971. p. 110.

50. Morse HN. Ritual circumcision. JAMA 1968 Mar 18;201(12): 256–8.

Holder AR. Circumcisions. JAMA 1971 Oct 4;218(1):149–50.

51. Associated Press. $1.4M awarded for botched circumcision. Santa Cruz Sentinel (9 June 2001): p. A5.

52. Fletcher CR. Circumcision in America in 1998: attitudes, beliefs, and charges of American physicians. In: Denniston GC, Hodges FM, Milos MF (eds). Male and Female Circumcision: Medical, Legal, and Ethical Considerations in Pediatric Practice. New York: Kluwer Academic/Plenum Publishers; 1999. pp. 259–71.

53. Mansfield CJ, Hueston WJ, Rudy M. Neonatal circumcision: associated factors and length of hospital stay. J Fam Pract 1995 Oct;41(4):370–6.

54. Bollinger D. Intact versus circumcised: male neonatal genital ratio in the United States. Circumcision Reference Library. 13 November 2000. URL: http://www.cirp.org/library/statistics/bollinger3/

55. Pitta J. Biosynthetics. Forbes (10 May 1993): pp. 170–1.

56. Arnst C. Science and Technology. The latest from the labs: human skin: the FDA is about to approve commercial use of living tissue grown by two biotech outfits. Business Week (18 May 1998): pp. 118–22.

57. Reuters. FDA approves human skin product to heal wounds. (29 May 1998). URL: http://www.sexuallymutilatedchild.org/f4sale.htm

58. Thompson HC, King LR, Knox E, Korones SB. Report of the ad hoc task force on circumcision. Pediatrics 1975 Oct;56(4):610–1.

59. Editor. Surgical mistake leads to lawsuit, sex-change operation on black baby. Jet 1985 Nov 25;69(11):29.

60. Editor. Botched circumcision costs Atlanta hospital $22.8 million. Jet 1991 Apr 1;79(25):9.

61. Morgan WKC. The rape of the phallus. JAMA 1965 Jul 19;193(3):223–4.

Preston EN. Whither the foreskin? A consideration of routine neonatal circumcision. JAMA 1970 Sep 14;213(11):1853–8.

Grimes DA. Routine circumcision of the newborn infant: a reappraisal. Am J Obstet Gynecol 1978 Jan 15;130(2):125–9.

62. Wiswell TE, Smith FR, Bass JW. Decreased incidence of urinary tract infections in circumcised male infants. Pediatrics 1985 May;75(5): 901–3.

63. Fink AJ. A possible explanation for heterosexual male infection with AIDS. N Engl J Med 1986 Oct 30;315(18):1167.

64. Weiss GN, Sanders M, Westbrook KC. The distribution and density of Langerhans cells in the human prepuce: site of a diminished immune response? Isr J Med Sci 1993 Jan;29(1):42–3.

65. Dagher R, Selzer ML, Lapides J. Carcinoma of the penis and the anti-circumcision crusade. J Urol 1973 Jul;110(1):79–80.

66. Ahmann S. Academy holds fast to position on circumcision. Pediatric News 1986 Sep;20(9):3, 38–9.

67. Schoen EJ. "Ode to the circumcised male." Am J Dis Child 1987 Feb;141(2):128.

Schoen EJ, Fischell AA. Dorsal penile nerve block for circumcision. JAMA 1989 Feb 3;261(5):701–2.

68. American Academy of Pediatrics: report of the Task Force on Circumcision. Pediatrics 1989 Aug;84(2):388–91.

69. Taylor JR, Lockwood AP, Taylor AJ. The prepuce: specialized mucosa of the penis and its loss to circumcision. Br J Urol 1996 Feb;77(2):291–5.

70. Australian College of Paediatrics. Position statement: routine circumcision of normal male infants and boys. Australian College of Paediatrics. 27 May 1996.

Fetus and Newborn Committee, Canadian Paediatric Society. Neonatal circumcision revisited. CMAJ 1996 Mar 15;154(6):769–80.

71. Task Force on Circumcision. Circumcision policy statement. American Academy of Pediatrics. Pediatrics 1999 Mar;103(3):686–93.

72. National Center for Health Statistics. Trends in Circumcisions Among Newborns. Hyattsville, MD: US Department of Health and Human Services. 18 July 2001. URL:http://www.cdc.gov/nchs/products/pubs/pubd/ hestats/circumcisions/circumcision.htm

Chapter 8: Are There Medical Benefits to Routine Circumcision?

1. Szasz T. Routine neonatal circumcision: symbol of the birth of the therapeutic state. J Med Philos 1996 Apr;21(2):137–48.

2. Campbell MF. The male genital tract and the female urethra. In: Campbell MF, Harrison JH, eds. Urology. 3rd ed. 3 vols. Philadelphia: W. B. Saunders Company; 1970. vol. 2. p. 1836.

Fishbein M. Sexual hygiene. In: Fishbein M (ed). Modern Home Medical Adviser. Garden City, NY: Doubleday & Company; 1969. p. 90.

3. American Academy of Pediatrics: Task Force on Circumcision. Circumcision policy statement. Pediatrics 1999 Mar;103(3):686–93.

4. Wolbarst AL. Circumcision and penile cancer. Lancet 1932 Jan 16;1(5655):150–3.

5. Wolbarst AL. Universal circumcision as a sanitary measure. JAMA 1914 Jan 10;62(2):92–7.

6. Ravich A. The relationship of circumcision to cancer of the prostate. J Urol 1942 Sep;48(3):298–9.

7. Ravich A, Ravich RA. Prophylaxis of cancer of the prostate, penis, and cervix by circumcision. NY State J Med 1951 Jun 15;51(12):1519–20.

8. Reddy G, Baruah IKSM. Carcinogenic action of human smegma. Arch Pathol 1963 Apr;75(4):414–20.

Pratt-Thomas HR, Heins HC, Latham E, Dennis EJ, McIver FA. The carcinogenic effect of human smegma: an experimental study. Cancer 1956 Jul–Aug;9(4):671–80.

Sobel H, Plaut A. The assimilation of cholesterol by mycobacterium smegmatis. J Bacteriol 1949 Mar;57(3):377–82.

9. Wright J. How smegma serves the penis. Sexology 1970 Sep;37(2):50–3.

10. Cutler SJ, Young JL Jr. Third national cancer survey: incidence data. Bethesda, MD. US Dept of Health, Education, and Welfare, Public Health Service.1975.

11. Frisch M, Friis S, Kjaer SK, Melbye M. Falling incidence of penis cancer in an uncircumcised population (Denmark, 1943–90). BMJ 1995 Dec 2;311(7018):1471.

12. Maiche AG. Epidemiological aspect of cancer of the penis in Finland. Eur J Cancer Prev 1992 Feb;1(2):153–8.

13. Cendron M, Elder JS, Duckett JW. Perinatal urology. In: Campbell's

Urology. 7th ed. vol. 3. Philadelphia: W. B. Saunders Company; 1998. p. 2151.

14. Maden C, Sherman KJ, Beckmann AM, Hislop TG, Teh C-Z, Ashley RL, Daling JR. History of circumcision, medical conditions, and sexual activity and risk of penile cancer. J Ntl Cancer Inst 1993 Jan 6;85(1):19–24.

15. Harish K, Ravi R. The role of tobacco in penile carcinoma. Br J Urol 1995 Mar;75(3):375–7.

Hellberg D, Valentin J, Eklund T, Nilsson S. Penile cancer: is there an epidemiological role for smoking and sexual behaviour? BMJ 1987 Nov 21;295(6609):1306–8.

16. Malek RS, Goellner JR, Smith TF, Espy MJ, Cupp MR. Human papillomavirus infection and intraepithelial, in situ and invasive carcinoma of the penis. Urology 1993 Aug;42(2):159–70.

17. Cupp MR, Malek RS, Goellner JR, Smith TF, Espey MJ. The detection of human papillomavirus deoxyribonucleic acid in intraepithelial, in situ, verrucous and invasive carcinoma of the penis. J Urol 1995 Sep;154(3):1024–9.

18. Wade TR, Kopf AW, Ackerman AB. Bowenoid papulosis of the penis. Cancer 1978 Oct;42(4):1890–903.

19. Tseng HF, Morgenstern, MT, Peters RK. Risk factors for penile cancer: results of a population-based case-control study in Los Angeles County (United States). Cancer Causes Control 2001 Apr;12(3):267–77.

20. Wiswell TE, Smith FR, Bass JW. Decreased incidence of urinary tract infections in circumcised male infants. Pediatrics 1985 May;75(5):901–3.

21. Gothefors L, Olling S, Winberg J. Breast feeding and biological properties of faecal E. coli strains. Acta Paediatr Scand 1975 Nov;54(6):807–12.

Winberg J, Gothefors L, Bollgren I, Herthelius M. The prepuce: a mistake of nature? Lancet 1989;1(8638):598–9.

Coppa GV, Gabrielli O, Giorgi P, Catassi C, Montanari MP, Varaldo PE, Nichols BL. Preliminary study of breastfeeding and bacterial adhesion to uroepithelial cells. Lancet 1990 Mar 10;335(8689):569–71.

Pisacane A, Graziano L, Zona G. Breastfeeding and urinary tract infection. Lancet 1990 Jul 7;336(8706):50.

Pisacane A, Graziano L, Mazzarella G, Scarpellino B, Zona G. Breastfeeding and urinary tract infection. J Pediatr 1992 Jan;120(1):87–9.

22. To T, Agha M, Dick PT, Feldman W. Cohort study on circumcision

of newborn boys and subsequent risk of urinary-tract infection. Lancet 1998 Dec 5;352(9143):1813–6.

23. Mueller ER, Steinhardt G, Naseer S. The incidence of genitourinary abnormalities in circumcised and uncircumcised boys presenting with an initial urinary tract infection by 6 months of age. Pediatrics 1997 Sep;100(3) Suppl:580.

24. Hand EA. Circumcision and venereal disease. Archives of Dermatology and Syphilology 1949 Sep;60(3):341–6.

25. Heimoff LL. Venereal disease control program. Bull US Army Med Dept 1945 Apr;3(87):93–100.

26. Smith GL, Greenup R, Takafuji ET. Circumcision as a risk factor for urethritis in racial groups. Am J Public Health 1987 Apr;77(4):452–4.

27. Donovan B, Bassett I, Bodsworth NJ. Male circumcision and common sexually transmissible diseases in a developed nation setting. Genitourin Med 1994 Oct;70(5):317–20.

28. Bassett I, Donovan B, Bodsworth NJ, Field PR, Ho DW, Jeansson S, Cunningham AL. Herpes simplex virus type 2 infection of heterosexual men attending a sexual health centre. Med J Aust 1994 Jun 6:160(11);697–700.

29. Cook LS, Koutsky LA, Holmes KK. Clinical presentation of genital warts among circumcised and uncircumcised heterosexual men attending an urban STD clinic. Genitourin Med 1993 Aug;69(4):262–4.

30. Van Howe RS. Does circumcision influence sexually transmitted diseases?: a literature review. BJU Int 1999 Jan;83 Suppl 1:52–62.

31. Laumann EO, Masi CM, Zuckerman EW. Circumcision in the United States: prevalence, prophylactic effects, and sexual practice. JAMA 1997 Apr 2;277(13):1052–7.

32. Fink AJ. A possible explanation for heterosexual male infection with AIDS. N Engl J Med 1986 Oct 30;315(18):1167.

33. Hand EA. Circumcision and venereal disease. Archives of Dermatology and Syphilology 1949 Sep;60(3):341–6.

34. Schoen EJ, Wiswell TE, Moses S. New policy on circumcision—cause for concern. Pediatrics 2000 Mar;105(3):620–3.

Schoen EJ. Is circumcision health? Yes. Priorities 1997 Winter;9(4):24, 26, 28.

35. Report on the Global HIV/AIDS Epidemic. June 2000 UNAIDS, Geneva, 2000, pp. 124–132. URL: www.unaids.org/epidemic_update/report/Epi_report.htm

36. Grulich AE, Hendry O, Clark E, Kippax S, Kaldor JM. Circumcision and male-to-male sexual transmission of HIV. AIDS 2001 Jun 15;15(9):1188–9.

37. Moses S, Bradley JE, Nagelkerke NJ, Ronald AR, Ndinya-Achola JO, Plummer FA. Geographical patterns of male circumcision practices in Africa: association with HIV seroprevalence. Int J Epidemiol 1990 Sep; 19(3):693–7.

38. Simonsen JN, Cameron DW, Gakinya MN, Ndinya-Achola JO, D'Costa LJ, Karasira P, Cheang M, Ronald AR, Piot P, Plummer FA. Human immunodeficiency virus infection among men with sexually transmitted diseases: experience from a center in Africa. N Engl J Med 1988 Aug 4;319(5):274–8.

Cameron DW, Simonsen JN, D'Costa LJ, Ronald AR, Maitha GM, Gakinya MN, Cheang M, Ndinya-Achola JO, Piot P, Brunham RC, et al. Female to male transmission of human immunodeficiency virus type 1: risk factors for seroconversion in men. Lancet 1989 Aug 19;2(8660):403–7.

Bwayo J, Plummer F, Omari M, Mutere A, Moses S, Ndinya-Achola J, Velentgas P, Kreiss J. Human immunodeficiency virus infection in long-distance truck drivers in east Africa. Arch Intern Med 1994 Jun 27;154(12):1391–6.

Bwayo JJ, Omari AM, Mutere AN, Jaoko W, Sekkade-Kigondu C, Kreiss J, Plummer FA. Long distance truck-drivers: 1. Prevalence of sexually transmitted diseases (STDs). East Afr Med J 1991 Jun;68(6):425–9.

Moses S, Plummer FA, Bradley JE, Ndinya-Achola JO, Nagelkerke NJ, Ronald AR. The association between lack of male circumcision and risk for HIV infection: a review of the epidemiological data. Sex Transm Dis 1994 Jul–Aug;21(4):201–10.

39. Laumann EO, Masi CM, Zuckerman EW. Circumcision in the United States: prevalence, prophylactic effects, and sexual practice. JAMA 1997 Apr 2;277(13):1052–7.

40. Runganga A, Pitts M, McMaster J. The use of herbal and other agents to enhance sexual experience. Soc Sci Med 1992 Oct;35(8):1037–42.

Runganga AO, Kasule J. The vaginal use of herbs/substances; an HIV transmission facilitatory factor? AIDS Care 1995;7(5):639–45.

Sandala L, Lurie P, Sunkutu MR, Chani EM, Hudes ES, Hearst N. "Dry sex" and HIV infection among women attending a sexually transmitted diseases clinic in Lusaka, Zambia. AIDS 1995 Jul;9 Suppl 1:S61–8.

Brown JE, Ayowa OB, Brown RC. Dry and tight: sexual practices and potential AIDS risk in Zaire. Soc Sci Med 1993 Oct;37(8):989–94.

Dallabetta GA, Miotti PG, Chiphangwi JD, Liomba G, Canner JK, Saah AJ. Traditional vaginal agents: use and association with HIV infection in Malawian women. AIDS 1995 Mar;9(3):293–7.

Gresenguet G, Kriess JK, Chapko MK, Hillier SL, Weiss NS. HIV infection and vaginal douching in central Africa. AIDS 1997 Jan;11(1):101–6.

Baleta A. Concern voiced over "dry sex" practices in South Africa. Lancet 1998 Oct 17;352(9136):1292.

Beksinska ME, Rees HV, Kleinschmidt I, McIntyre J. The practice and prevalence of dry sex among men and women in South Africa: a risk factor for sexually transmitted infections? Sex Transm Infect 1999 Jun;75(3): 178–80.

41. Pepin J, Quigley M, Todd J, Gaye I, Janneh M, Van Dyck E, Piot P, Whittle H. Association between HIV-2 infection and genital ulcer diseases among male sexually transmitted disease patients in the Gambia. AIDS 1992 May;6(5):489–93.

O'Farrell N, Hoosen AA, Coetzee KD, van den Ende J. Sexual behaviour in Zulu men and women with genital ulcer disease. Genitourin Med 1992 Aug;68(4):245–8.

de Vincenzi I, Mertens T. Male circumcision: a role in HIV prevention? AIDS 1994 Feb;8(2):153–60.

42. O'Farrell N, Hoosen AA, Coetzee KD, van den Ende J. Sexual behaviour in Zulu men and women with genital ulcer disease. Genitourin Med 1992 Aug;68(4):245–8.

43. Kaul R, Kimani J, Nagelkerke NJ, Plummer FA, Bwayo JJ, Brunham RC, Ngugi EN, Ronald A. Risk factors for genital ulcerations in Kenyan sex workers: the role of human immunodeficiency virus type 1 infection. Sex Transm Dis 1997 Aug;24(7):387–92.

44. Hrdy DB. Cultural practices contributing to the transmission of human immunodeficiency virus in Africa. Rev Infect Dis 1987 Nov–Dec;9(6):1109–19.

Brady M. Female genital mutilation: complications and risk of HIV transmission. AIDS Patient Care STDS 1999 Dec;13(12):709–16.

45. Quinn TC, Wawer MJ, Sewankambo N, Serwadda D, Li C, Wabwire-Mangen F, Meehan MO, Lutalo T, Gray RH. Viral load and heterosexual transmission of human immunodeficiency virus type 1. Rakai Project Study Group. N Engl J Med 2000 Mar 30;342(13):921–9.

46. Peiperl L. The Rakai study: risk factors for heterosexual transmission. InSite Journal Club. 14 April 2000. URL: http://hivinsite.ucsf.edu/medical/journal_club/2098.46f3.html

47. Kelly R, Kiwanuka N, Wawer MJ, Serwadda D, Sewankambo NK, Wabwire-Mangen F, Li C, Konde-Lule JK, Lutalo T, Makumbi F, Gray RH. Age of male circumcision and risk of prevalent HIV infection in rural Uganda. AIDS 1999 Feb 25;13(3):399–405.

48. Parkash S, Rao R, Venkatesan K, Ramafrishnan S. Sub-preputial wetness—its nature. Ann Natl Med Sci (India) 1982 Jul–Sep;18(3):109–12.

49. Lee-Huang S, Huang PL, Sun Y, Huang PL, Kung HF, Blithe DL, Chen HC. Lysozyme and RNases as anti-HIV components in beta-core preparations of human chorionic gonadotropin. Proc Natl Acad Sci USA 1999 Mar 16;96(6):2678–81.

50. American Academy of Pediatrics. Task Force on Circumcision. Circumcision policy statement. Pediatrics 1999 Mar;103(3):686–93.

51. Council on Scientific Affairs, American Medical Association. Neonatal circumcision (Report 10). Chicago: American Medical Association; 2000.

52. VanHowe RS. Variability in penile appearance and penile findings: a prospective study. Br J Urol 1997 Nov;80(5):776–82.

53. Oster J. Further fate of the foreskin: incidence of preputial adhesions, phimosis, and smegma among Danish schoolboys. Arch Dis Child 1968 Apr;43(228):200–3.

54. Reimbursement adviser. How to get reimbursed for circumcision. OBG Management 1993 Oct;5(3):25.

55. Oster J. Further fate of the foreskin: incidence of preputial adhesions, phimosis, and smegma among Danish schoolboys. Arch Dis Child 1968 Apr;43(228):200–3.

Kayaba H, Tamura H, Kitajima S, Fujiwara Y, Kato T, Kato T. Analysis of shape and retractability of the prepuce in 603 Japanese boys. J Urol 1996 Nov;156(5):1813–5.

56. Rickwood AM. Medical indications for circumcision. BJU Int 1999 Jan;83 Suppl 1:45–51.

Shankar KR, Rickwood AM. The incidence of phimosis in boys. BJU Int 1999 Jul;84(1):101–2.

Rickwood AM, Kenny SE, Donnell SC. Towards evidence based circumcision of English boys: survey of trends in practice. BMJ 2000 Sep 30;321(7264):792–3.

57. Jorgensen ET, Svensson A. The treatment of phimosis in boys, with a potent topical steroid (clobetasol propionate 0.05%) cream. Acta Derm Verereol 1993 Feb;73(1):55–6.

Van Howe RS. Cost-effective treatment of phimosis. Pediatrics 1998 Oct;102(4):E43.

Lindhagen T. Topical clobetasol propionate compared with placebo in the treatment of unretractable foreskin. Eur J Surg 1996 Dec;162(12): 969–72.

Berdeu D, Sauze L, Ha-Vinh P, Blum-Boisgard C. Cost-effectiveness analysis of treatments for phimosis: a comparison of surgical and medicinal approaches and their economic effect. BJU Int 2001 Feb;87(3):239–44.

58. Cuckow PM, Rix G, Mouriquand PDE. Preputial plasty: a good alternative to circumcision. J Pediatr 1994 Apr;29(4):561–3.

Wahlin N. "Triple incision plasty": a convenient procedure for preputial relief. Scand J Urol Nephrol 1992;26(2):107–10.

Pascotto R, Giancotti E. [The treatment of phimosis in childhood without circumcision: plastic repair of the prepuce]. Minerva Chir 1998 Jun;53(6):561–5.

59. Beaugé M. Traitement médical du phimosis congénital de l'adolescent. Thèse de Paris (Faculté de Médecine, Saint-Antoine Université Paris VI). 1990.

60. Ravich A, Ravich R A. Prophylaxis of cancer of the prostate, penis, and cervix by circumcision. NY State Med 1951 Jun;51(12):1519–20.

61. Wynder EL, Cornfield J, Schroff PD, Doraiswami KR. A Study of Environmental Factors in Carcinoma of the Cervix. Am J Obstet Gynecol 1954 Oct;68(4):1016–52.

62. Editor. Circumcision and cancer. Time 1954 Apr 5;63(14):96–7.

63. Lilienfeld AM, Graham S. Validity of determining circumcision status by questionnaire as related to epidemiological studies of cancer of the cervix. J Ntl Cancer Inst 1958 Oct;21(4):713–20.

64. Wynder EL, Licklider SD. The question of circumcision. Cancer 1960 May–Jun;13(3):442–5.

65. Wynder EL, Mantel N, Licklider SD. Statistical considerations on circumcision and cervical cancer. Am J Obstet Gynecol 1960 May;79(5): 1026–30.

66. Jones EG, MacDonald I, Breslow L. A study of epidemiologic factors in carcinoma of the uterine cervix. Am J Obstet Gynecol 1958 Jul;76(1):1–10.

Stern E, Dixon WJ. Cancer of the cervix: a biometric approach to etiology. Cancer 1961 Jan–Feb;14(1):153–60.

Aitken-Swan J, Baird D. Circumcision and cancer of the cervix. Br J Cancer 1965 Jun;19(2):217–27.

Abou-Daoud-KT. Epidemiology of carcinoma of the cervix uteri in Lebanese Christians and Moslems. Cancer 1967 Oct;20(10):1706–14.

Stern E, Lachenbruch PA. Circumcision information in a cancer detection center population. J Chronic Dis 1968 May;21(2):117–24.

Christopherson WM. The geographic distribution of cervix cancer and its possible implications. J Ir Med Assoc 1968 Jan;61(367):1–3.

Malhotra SL. A study of carcinoma of uterine cervix with special reference to its causation and prevention. Br J Cancer 1971 Mar;25(1):62–71.

Terris M, Wilson F, Nelson JH Jr. Relation of circumcision to cancer of the cervix. Am J Obstet Gynecol 1973 Dec 15;117(8):1056–66.

Alexander ER. Possible etiologies of cancer of the cervix other than herpesvirus. Cancer Res 1973 Jun;33(6):1485–90.

Harington JS. Epidemiology and aetiology of cancer of the uterine cervix including the detection of carcinogenic N-nitrosamines in the human vaginal vault. S Afr Med J 1975 Mar 19;49(12):443–5.

Persaud V. Geographical pathology of cancer of the uterine cervix. Trop Geogr Med 1977 Dec;29(4):335–45.

Sumithran E. Rarity of cancer of the cervix in the Malaysian Orang Asli despite the presence of known risk factors. Cancer 1977 Apr;39(4):1570–2.

Naik KG. Cervical carcinoma in Zambia. Int Surg 1977 Feb;62(2):110–1.

Megafu U. Cancer of the genital tract among the Ibo women in Nigeria. Cancer 1979 Nov;44(5):1875–8.

Lee JP, Cuello C, Singh K. Review of the epidemiology of cervical cancer in the Pacific Basin. Natl Cancer Inst Monogr 1982;62:197–9.

Brinton LA, Reeves WC, Brenes MM, Herrero R, Gaitan E, Tenorio F, de-Britton RC, Garcia M, Rawls WE. The male factor in the etiology of cervical cancer among sexually monogamous women. Int J Cancer 1989 Aug 15;44(2):199–203.

67. Spock B. Notes on the psychology of circumcision, masturbation and enuresis. Urologic and Cutaneous Review 1942 Dec;46(12):768–70.

Chapter 9: Common Nonmedical Excuses for Routine Circumcision

1. Goldman R. The psychological impact of circumcision. BJU Int 1999 Jan;83:93–102.

2. Brown MS, Brown CA. Circumcision decision: prominence of social concerns. Pediatrics 1987 Aug;80(2):215–9.

Herrera AJ, Hsu AS, Salcedo UT, Ruiz MP. The role of parental information in the incidence of circumcision. Pediatrics 1982 Oct;70(4):597–8.

Herrera AJ, Cochran B, Herrera A, Wallace B. Parental information and circumcision in highly motivated couples with higher education. Pediatrics 1983 Feb;71(2):233–4.

Chapter 10: Most Common Reasons Given for Postneonatal Circumcision

1. Leboyer F. Personal correspondence to Rosemary Romberg, 4 June 1980. Reproduced in: Romberg R. Circumcision: The Painful Dilemma. South Hadley, Mass: Bergin & Garvey Publishers; 1985. p. vii.

2. Birley HD, Walker MM, Luzzi GA, Bell R, Taylor-Robinson D, Byrne M, Renton AM. Clinical features and management of recurrent balanitis; association with atopy and genital washing. Genitourin Med 1993 Oct;69(5):400–3.

3. Taylor JR, Lockwood AP, Taylor AJ. The prepuce: specialized mucosa of the penis and its loss to circumcision. Br J Urol 1996 Feb;77(2):291–5.

Cold CJ, Taylor JR. The prepuce. BJU Int 1999 Jan;83 Suppl 1:34–44.

4. Anand KJ, Hickey PR. Pain and its effects in the human neonate and fetus. N Engl J Med 1987 Nov 19;317(21):1321–9.

5. Garry T. Circumcision: a survey of fees and practices. OBG Management (October) 1994:34–36.

Stang HJ, Snellman LW. Circumcision practice patterns in the United States. Pediatrics 1998 Jun;101(6):E5.

Howard CR, Howard FM, Garfunkel LC, de Blieck EA, Weitzman M. Neonatal circumcision and pain relief: current training practices. Pediatrics 1998 Mar;101(3 Pt 1):423–8.

6. Hillhollon M. Patient for heart bypass sues over circumcision. Advocate ONLINE (Baton Rouge, Louisiana), (17 March 2000): URL: http:/www.theadvocate.com/news/story/asp?StoryID=1165

7. Winberg J, Bollgren I, Gothefors L, Herthelius M, Tullus K. The prepuce: a mistake of nature? Lancet 1989 Mar 18;1(8638):598–9.

Downs SM. Technical report: urinary tract infections in febrile infants and young children. The Urinary Tract Subcommittee of the American Academy of Pediatrics Committee on Quality Improvement. Pediatrics 1999 Apr;103(4):e54.

Gill MA, Schutze GE. Citrobacter urinary tract infections in children. Pediatr Infect Dis J 1999 Oct;18(10):889–92.

8. Nolan JF, Stillwell TJ, Sands JP Jr. Acute management of the zipper-entrapped penis. J Emerg Med 1990 May–Jun;8(3):305–7.

Oosterlinck W. Unbloody management of penile zipper injury. Eur Urol 1981;7(6):365–6.

Flowerdew R, Fishman IJ, Churchill BM. Management of penile zipper injury. J Urol 1977 May;117(5):671.

9. Kanegaye JT, Schonfeld N. Penile zipper entrapment: a simple and less threatening approach using mineral oil. Pediatr Emerg Care 1993 Apr;9(2):90–1.

10. Houghton GR. The "ice-glove" method of treatment of paraphimosis. Br J Surg 1973 Nov;60(11):876–7.

DeVries CR, Miller AK, Packer MG. Reduction of paraphimosis with hyaluronidase. Urology 1996 Sep;48(3):464–5.

11. Kerwat R, Shandall A, Stephenson B. Reduction of paraphimosis with granulated sugar. Br J Urol 1998 Nov;82(5):755.

12. Reynard JM, Barua JM. Reduction of paraphimosis the simple way—the Dundee technique. BJU Int 1999 May;83(7):859–60.

13. Jorgensen ET, Svensson A. The treatment of phimosis in boys, with a potent topical steroid (clobetasol propionate 0.05%) cream. Acta Derm Venereol 1993 Feb;73(1):55–6.

Van Howe RS. Cost-effective treatment of phimosis. Pediatrics 1998 Oct;102(4):E43.

Lindhagen T. Topical clobetasol propionate compared with placebo in the treatment of unretractable foreskin. Eur J Surg 1996 Dec; 162(12):969–72.

Berdeu D, Sauze L, Ha-Vinh P, Blum-Boisgard C. Cost-effectiveness analysis of treatments for phimosis: a comparison of surgical and medicinal approaches and their economic effect. BJU Int 2001 Feb;87(3):239–44.

14. Ratz JL. Carbon dioxide laser treatment of balanitis xerotica obliterans. J Am Acad Dermatol 1984 May;10(5 Pt 2):925–8.

Rosemberg SK, Jacobs H. Continuous wave carbon dioxide treatment of balanitis xerotica obliterans. Urology 1982 May;19(5):539–41.

Hrebinko RL. Circumferential laser vaporization for severe meatal stenosis secondary to balanitis xerotica obliterans. J Urol 1996 Nov;156(5):1735–6.

Windahl T, Hellsten S. Carbon dioxide laser treatment of lichen sclerosus et atrophicus. J Urol 1993 Sep;150(3):868–70.

Kartamaa M, Reitamo S. Treatment of lichen sclerosus with carbon dioxide laser vaporization. Br J Dermatol 1997 Mar;136(3):356–9.

15. Shelley WB, Shelley ED, Grunenwald MA, Anders TJ, Ramnath A. Long-term antibiotic therapy for balanitis xerotica obliterans. J Am Acad Dermatol 1999 Jan;40(1):69–72.

16. Cuckow PM, Rix G, Mouriquand PDE. Preputial plasty: a good alternative to circumcision. J Pediatr 1994 Apr;29(4):561–3.

Wahlin N. "Triple incision plasty": a convenient procedure for preputial relief. Scand J Urol Nephrol 1992;26(2):107–10.

Pascotto R, Giancotti E. [The treatment of phimosis in childhood without circumcision: plastic repair of the prepuce]. Minerva Chir 1998 Jun;53(6):561–5.

Chapter 11: The Care of Your Son's Intact Penis

1. Erickson JA. Cited in: Answers to Your Questions About Your Son's Intact Penis. National Organization of Circumcision Information Resource Centers. Nov. 1997. www.nocirc.org

2. American Academy of Pediatrics. Care of the Uncircumcised Penis. Evanston, Ill: American Academy of Pediatrics; 1984.

Chapter 12: Care of the Circumcised Penis

1. Koop CE. Dr. Koop on circumcision. Saturday Evening Post 1982 Jul–Aug;254(5):6.

2. Macke JK. Analgesia for circumcision: effects on newborn behavior and mother/infant interaction. J Obstet Gynecol Neonatal Nurs 2001 Sep–Oct;30(5):507–14.

3. Taylor JR, Lockwood AP, Taylor AJ. The prepuce: specialized mucosa of the penis and its loss to circumcision. Br J Urol 1996 Feb;77(2):291–5.

Chapter 13: Afterthoughts

1. Economic Justice for All. Pastoral Letter on Catholic Social Teaching and the U.S. Economy. U.S. Catholic Bishops, 1986. URL: http://www.osjspm.org/cst/eja.htm

Appendix A

1. American Medical Association. Report 10 of the Council on Scientific Affairs (I-99). Neonatal Circumcision. 6 July 2000. URL: http://www.nocirc.org/

2. American Academy of Pediatrics. Task Force on Circumcision. Circumcision Policy Statement. Pediatrics 1999 Mar;103(3):686–93.

3. American College of Obstetricians and Gynecologists. Committee on Obstetric Practice. ACOG Committee Opinion. Circumcision. No. 260, October 2001. Obstet Gynecol 2001 Oct;98(4):707–8.

4. Hugh Shingleton, M.D., National Vice President Detection & Treatment; Clark W. Heath, Jr., M.D. Vice President Epidemiology & Surveillance Research. American Cancer Society. Letter to Dr. Peter Rappo. Committee on Practice & Ambulatory Medicine American Academy of Pediatrics. 16 February 1996. Letter available for inspection at URL: http://www.nocirc.org/

5. Leditschke JF. The Australasian Association of Paediatric Surgeons. Guidelines for Circumcision. April 1996. URL: http://www.nocirc.org/

6. The Australian College of Paediatrics. Position Statement. Routine Circumcision of Normal Male Infants and Boys. 27 May 1996. URL: http://www.nocirc.org/

7. British Medical Association. Circumcision of Male Infants: Guidance for Doctors. September 1996. URL: http://www.nocirc.org/

8. Fetus and Newborn Committee, Canadian Paediatric Society. Neonatal circumcision revisited. Can Med Assoc J 1996 Mar 15;153(6):769–80.

Index

abdominal distension, 61
Abraham, 102, 117
Abu-Sahlieh, Dr. S. A. Aldeeb, 114
acidophilus, 197
adhesions, 71, 221
adult circumcision, 68, 74, 200–201
Advanced Tissue Sciences, 141–142
Africa
  circumcision in, xv, 92, 114–115,
    119–120
  HIV in, 160, 161–166
African Americans. *See* blacks; racism
AIDS. *See* HIV
akroposthion, 3–4, 7
alcohol, as anesthesia, 46
alcoholism, 152
Alexander the Great, 120
AlloDerm, 141
Ambrose, St., 99–100
American Academy of Pediatrics (AAP)
  on anesthesia, 46–47
  on circumcision in delivery room, 68
  on HIV infection, 166
  on routine circumcision, 111, 137,
    142, 144–145, 149–150
  on UTIs, 155

American Medical Association (AMA),
    166–167
anal intercourse, 161, 164
anesthesia
  absence of, during circumcision, 37,
    39, 43, 46–47, 114, 132, 200, 216
  complications from, 64–66, 74, 218
  creams, 64–65
  dangers of, 47, 59
  infiltrative, 65
anorexia, 69
antibiotics, 154–155, 177, 202, 206
Antiochus IV Epiphanes, 120
apes, foreskin and glans of, 15
apnea, 43, 57, 66–67
apocrine glands, 21
Apostolical Canons of the Church, 98–99
appendectomy, 200
appendix, function of, 15
Arabs. *See* Muslims
Augustine, St., 99
Australia, xv, 161
Australian College of Paediatrics, 145

bacteremia, 55
bacteria, 22, 55, 57, 166

ABOUT THE AUTHORS

Paul M. Fleiss, MD, MPH, FAAP, is a well-respected pediatrician who has been in practice for over thirty-five years. In that time, he has cared for a generation of children, many of whom now bring their own children to the California Craftsman bungalow that houses the Fleiss pediatric office. In addition to his medical degree, Dr. Fleiss has a Bachelor of Science degree in Pharmacy and a Master of Public Health degree. Paul Fleiss has been well published in his impressive career in publications as wide ranging as *The Journal of the American Medical Association* to *Mothering* magazine. He has given numerous presentations over the years on topics from breast-feeding to the use of herbal remedies. He has also received several research grants to study the excretion of pharmaceutical drugs in human milk. He maintains an active medical practice in Los Angeles.

Frederick Mansfield Hodges, D.Phil, is a medical historian and author. He is currently a postdoctoral research associate in the Department of History at Yale University. After earning his Bachelor of Arts at the University of California at Berkeley, Dr. Hodges earned both his master's and his doctorate at the University of Oxford in England, under the aegis of its prestigious Wellcome Unit for the History of Medicine. His medical and historical research on a wide range of topics, from antiquity to the present, has been published in such journals as the *British Medical Journal,* the *Bulletin of the History of Medicine,* the *World Journal of Urology, Sexually Transmitted Diseases,* and *Pediatrics.* He has also given numerous presentations at medical conferences, including the annual meetings of the European Association of Urology, the World Congress of Urology, and the Royal College of Paediatrics and Child Health.